Get Fit While You Sit

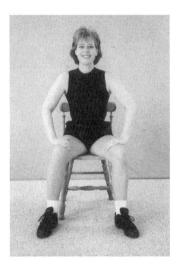

Dedication

To my husband, Tim, for his many patient hours behind the camera.

Ordering
Trade bookstores in the U.S. and Canada please contact:

Publishers Group West
1700 Fourth Street, Berkeley CA 94710
Phone: (800) 788-3123 Fax: (510) 528-3444

Hunter House books are available at bulk discounts for textbook course adoptions; to qualifying community, healthcare, and government organizations; and for special promotions and fundraising. For details please contact:

Special Sales Department
Hunter House Inc., PO Box 2914, Alameda CA 94501-0914
Tel. (510) 865-5282 Fax (510) 865-4295 e-mail: marketing@hunterhouse.com

Individuals can order our books from most bookstores or by calling toll-free:

1-800-266-5592

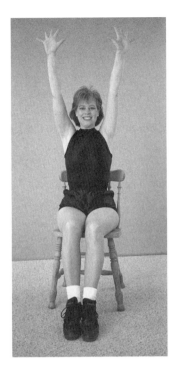

'GET FIT WHILE YOU SIT

Easy Workouts from Your Chair

by
Charlene Torkelson

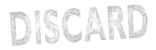

Hunter House
PUBLISHERS

    Hunter House Inc., Publishers
    PO Box 2914
    Alameda CA 94501-0914

Library of Congress Cataloging-in-Publication Data

Torkelson, Charlene.
    Get fit while you sit : easy workouts from your chair / Charlene Torkelson. — 1st ed.
       p.   cm.
    Includes bibliographical references.
    ISBN 0-89793-254-4 (hbk.). — ISBN 0-89793-253-6 (pbk.)
    1. Exercise. 2. Sitting position. I. Title.
RA781.T66 199
613.7'1—dc21   99-11982
                                                                      CIP

Project credits
Cover Design: Peri Poloni
Book Design and Production: Margaret Copeland, Terragraphics
Copy Editing: Priscilla Stuckey, Kiran Rana
Proofreader: Susan Burckhard
Managing Editor: Wendy Low
Editorial Coordinators: Jeanne Brondino, Jennifer Rader
Publicity: Marisa Spatafore
Marketing Intern: Monique Portegies
Customer Service Manager: Christina Sverdrup
Order Fulfillment: Joel Irons; A & A Quality Shipping Services
Publisher: Kiran S. Rana

Printed and bound by Publishers Press, Salt Lake City, UT
9 8 7 6 5 4 3 2 1   First Edition   99 00 01 02 03

Contents

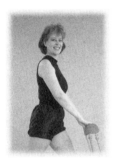
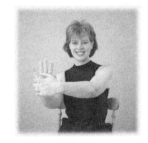

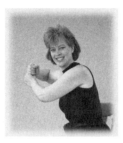

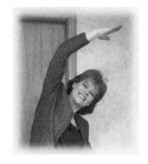

Acknowledgments

A special thank you to Maxine Vashro, who asked me to do this chair class in the first place. Thank you to the seniors in my chair classes from Robbinsdale Senior Center. They are the ones who inspired me to design this program and who gave me so much praise and support through their fitness results. Thanks to my photographer, Tim Torkelson; my photographic consultant, Craig Perman; my computer consultant, Tom La Tourelle; and my family, Beau, Breanna, and Luke. Thanks, Mom, Ruth Behrend, who has proudly showed my manuscript to anyone she felt would benefit from this program. Thank you to my medical adviser, Dr. Son Nguyen. Thank you to the people at Hunter House Publishers, especially Jeanne Brondino.

Disclaimer

The material in this book is intended to provide a safe, effective exercise program. However, the reader is advised to consult a physician before beginning any exercise program, especially any reader with pre-existing medical problems. As professionals in the field may have differing opinions and change is always taking place, the authors, publisher, and editors cannot be held responsible for any error, omission, dated material, or adverse outcomes that may result from using the information and exercises provided in this book in a program of self-care or under the care of a licensed practitioner.

Introduction

It has been a great pleasure to develop and teach my "chair class" at the Robbinsdale Senior Center. The popularity of the chair method with my students led me to realize that this program has potential for everyone. People need to be introduced to chair exercises for many reasons. We all sit, some of us much longer than is healthy for us. Also, chair exercises have the great benefit of being something we can do wherever we are. All we need is a chair. When the weather is too cold or wet for a walk or a trip to the health club, chair exercises can keep us fit. And for many, these low-impact, low-demand exercises are a safe and marvelous way to increase fitness with minimal expense.

To introduce the program, let's look at some frequently asked questions:

Who should try the chair fitness program?

This program is designed for everyone. Those who will find it most helpful are:

- People who have done little or no exercise for some time. Unfortunately, people who are not on an exercise program realize they should be but cannot fit easily into the existing programs. These programs are just too strenuous or too difficult. So after one or two attempts, they never go back. Many exercise programs are for those who are already very fit. Exercise need not be hard, and programs should encourage those who are not already in top shape. Consistency is the key to better fitness.

- People who work at a desk or travel frequently. When it is necessary to be seated for a great deal of time, it is wonderful to have an exercise program that fits into that situation. It relieves the boredom, tension, and stiffness caused by sitting.

- People who have physical or medical limitations. For whatever reason, these people may find traditional programs either uncomfortable or poorly suited to their needs. I always recommend that people with medical difficulties check with their physician before beginning an exercise program to be sure it meets those needs and limitations.

- People who feel uncoordinated, have difficulties with balance, or are uncomfortable in a conventional program for any reason. As we get older we find our balance is not what it used to be. I frequently hear people say to me, "I just can't get down on the floor anymore." Nor should they have to. Many seniors find our chair exercises an ideal program for their needs.

- Children also find this to be a great program. Children often feel uncertain about their sense of balance. They need a program that they can do easily without very complex or detailed directions. The chair program is one they can do in the home together with parents or other adults.

What are the benefits of a chair program?

If people find an exercise program easy, inexpensive, and fun, they will continue. The most important element of any exercise is *consistency*. Any exercise program is beneficial only if it is done consistently. Unfortunately for us, one strenuous bout with exercise does not last the year. Many people seem to think this way. They push themselves through one session, feel tired and sore for a few days, and then feel that will last them forever. It doesn't work that way.

We live in an age of inactivity. This is the era of the "Couch Potato." With television, videos, and computers so prevalent, most people spend a great deal of time sitting. So exercise becomes even more important.

Exactly how "easy, inexpensive, and fun" is this program?

Let's begin with *inexpensive*. A chair program needs basically only two elements—a chair, and weights.

The chair should not be a rocking chair or a big comfy soft chair—although some of the exercises may be done wherever you are. They can be done in your car during traffic jams or at your desk at work. The best chair is a straight-backed chair without arms. The arms can get in your way on some of the exercises.

That means you don't need to go to the gym or pay for a club membership. You don't need to find a court or a pool to get your exercise. You don't need to invest in expensive equipment that you don't have room for anyway. You can sit in your own living room. You can even exercise while you listen to the radio or watch TV. It doesn't have to be boring.

Some exercises do include small hand-held weights. These are relatively inexpensive and can be purchased in any department store. Most people spend two or three dollars per weight. We recommend purchasing one-, two-, or three-pound weights. Many people find the one pound too light and the three pound too heavy, so the most popular weight is the two pound. Use your discretion, and look at your own abilities and needs.

You don't even need to invest in weights if you don't choose to. You can lift soup cans or pop bottles filled with sand. You don't need to spend anything at all for your weights.

Now let's go to *easy*. As I've explained, some of the exercises are designed to be done anywhere. They can be done at the dinner table or at your desk at work. We call these exercises "isolations." That means we focus on a muscle, tightening and relaxing it. No one even has to know you are exercising.

With the chair program you don't need to spend money, go somewhere else, or dress in a special way. It is meant to be easy, so you will do it and continue to do it.

Now for *fun*. If you enjoy exercising to music, put on music. That always makes things more fun. And the really fun part of it is that you can choose any music you like. You can listen to classical, rock, rap, or gospel. Pick what you like, not what someone else chooses for you—and play it as loud as you like!

You can exercise at home with your family and friends, or when traveling. Use the exercises for relieving boredom on long car or bus trips, and for relaxing or relieving stiffness on airplane flights.

Remember, you are in charge. Exercise in the morning, over lunch, or in the evening.

Select a time that is convenient for you. You don't need to follow someone else's schedule. Put your exercise in where and when you choose. Invite a friend. Exercise with your dog. As you do, you'll notice yourself feeling better.

We all know that exercise is good for us. But we tend to put it off if we think it will be hard or inconvenient. New people in my class always say, "I think I can do this," after the first class. As they improve each week, they feel proud. In fact, they seem to glow with satisfaction. And they feel better physically, too.

Why do I need to exercise at all?

Today, almost everyone recognizes the importance of exercise. Not only does it improve physical health, it also improves mental and emotional health. If you could feel better and do something that is actually good for you, why wouldn't you do it? Especially when it is fun, easy, and inexpensive? What more could you ask for?

How do I get started?

First, select your chair. Pick a chair that is solid. It shouldn't rock back and forth or feel as if it will collapse. Also, as mentioned, your basic exercise chair shouldn't have arms, because they might interfere with some of the exercises.

Second, select your weights. You may purchase a pair of inexpensive weights or use something from your own kitchen.

Third, wear something loose and comfortable.

We have a standing joke in my class. People always seem to color-coordinate. Often, they wear something that matches the color of their weights. I always tell them how good they look—though it's hardly what you would expect someone about to exercise to be worrying about.

Fourth, if you like to have music in the background, select something you like. It makes exercise fun. Personally, I watch game shows on television when I exercise. Time goes so quickly.

Fifth, if you have a physical or medical condition, check with your doctor before you begin any exercise program.

Now, get out this book and copy as best you can the exercises pictured. I have tried to explain the exercise as well as demonstrate the proper position in the photographs. It is better to exercise properly than to do more, faster, and improper movements. You will find each time you do the exercises they become easier. As they become easier, feel free to add more repetitions.

I walk right now. Why should I do this program?

Walking is a wonderful exercise. That is why walking is included in this program as an aerobic exercise. In addition to walking, this program tries to encompass all the parts of the body. If you are like most people, you focus on the easiest part, ignoring exercises that don't feel as easy to do. But that might mean you are ignoring an important part of your body. I am very flexible, so I find leg exercises very easy. But I shy away from stomach exercises, because I don't enjoy them as much. So I have to concentrate more on my stomach exercises because I find them harder than the leg exercises.

This program does a little with every part of the body. Most people are especially pleased with the weights section, since we often neglect exercises that develop our arms and upper body strength.

The most fun section, though, is the relaxing cool-down at the end. Most of the people in my class are so relaxed at the end of class that they don't even feel as if they've exercised. Hopefully, you will feel the same way.

How often should I exercise?

That is up to you. Depending on your time and energy, you could exercise once, twice, or three times a week. You may even be the kind of person who enjoys it so much, you do some every day. Most agree that three times a week is ideal. But don't feel terrible if you don't have the time to do it that often. What's most important is to be consistent.

Some in my class begin with a once-a-week schedule. Many ask after a few weeks if they can increase to two or three times a week. They feel confident that they are able to do the exercises. You can do them as often as you would like and your schedule and fitness level allow.

My doctor advises me to do low-impact exercise. Does this qualify?

Yes. *Low-impact* refers to exercises that do not put undue stress on your joints—ankles, knees, and hips. When you jump and bounce, you can injure those joints. I myself always do low-impact exercise because of an old knee injury. Low-impact exercise is a much safer style of exercise.

If these exercises are easy, will they do anything for me?

People who look and feel fit are not necessarily people who exercise rigorously all the time. They are, instead, people who consistently put exercise into their lives. These exercises do not need to be strenuous. We seem to feel that if we aren't sore, it wasn't worthwhile. "No pain, no gain" is really an untruth. Doing easy exercises regularly will help keep you fit. And people who are fit walk more consistently. That doesn't mean they walk around the track a few miles each day. It may mean they park their car toward the back of the lot at the supermarket or walk up the stairs instead of taking the elevator. There are many little ways of keeping fit.

That is why this program is so great. It is little consistent things that make you look and feel more fit. Little things easily become a habit. So lots of little good habits add up

to a healthy exercise program that is easy and fun to follow.

In addition to a one-hour workout, I have included 10-minute workouts for those who have a limited time. There is a special chapter for those of you who are really rushed and need help with working a fitness program into your very hectic day. Chapter 4 also includes special exercises for the computer user who must spend extended periods of time sitting in one place.

If you have any special physical concerns, turn to Chapter 2 for additional advice. The areas covered include back, head and neck, legs and stomach areas, as well as additional exercises for those with arthritis and osteoporosis.

When you have gained a good foundation and understanding of the exercises you will naturally adopt a plan that you feel fits into your schedule and lifestyle. Then you can use the exercise charts provided at the back of the book to make your program even simpler to maintain.

Have fun!

Chapter 1

························

The One-Hour Chair Program

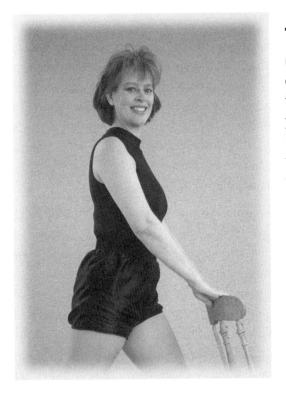

The one-hour chair program includes a warm-up, aerobic exercise in the form of walking, exercises with weights, and a cool-down. It takes approximately one hour to complete. If you find it too long because you are rushed or if it is too strenuous for you to begin with, turn to chapter 2, "Workouts for Special Conditions," or chapters 3 and 4, which give ten-minute exercise programs.

■ The Warm-Up

The warm-up is important. It prevents injury and allows our muscles to get used to exercising. This prevents us from feeling stiff and sore later. I recommended earlier that you add repetitions to your exercise program after you feel comfortable. This isn't necessary with the warm-up. The warm-up repetitions are used only to stretch out our muscles before we do the other exercises. Remember the three C's of exercise: exercise *carefully*, exercise *correctly*, and exercise *consistently*. We'll talk more about each of these throughout the book. For now, exercise correctly by carefully following the positions in each picture.

Deep Breathing

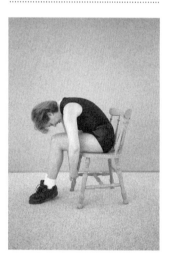

I always include breathing exercises in the warm-up and cool-down. Many people are shallow breathers. They take a short breath into the upper chest area. With the deep breathing exercises, we learn to breathe lower into the lungs so our abdomen muscles expand, too. This improves our circulation and helps our lungs and heart to function more comfortably. Breathing is an important exercise.

Sit on the edge of the chair so your arms don't hit the legs or edge of the chair. Feet should be positioned squarely on the floor and together. This keeps your posture straight. Start by exhaling and bending forward until your hands are below your knees. Now inhale, and raise your arms up over your head as you do. Then exhale, lowering your arms, until your hands are again at the position beneath your knees. I warm up with a few inhales/exhales (about 3 or 4). Then do this exercise holding your breath for a few seconds before exhaling. I recommend holding the inhale 3 times. Notice the starting and ending positions pictured below.

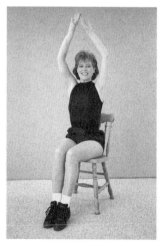

Overhead Stretch

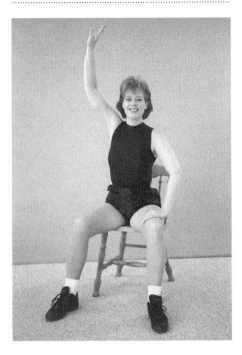

Sit with your feet flat on the floor and separated, to provide balance. Support your left hand on your left knee. Reach up with your right arm and stretch it straight above your head. Turn your palm over as if you were going to wash the ceiling, and lean over toward your left side. Your right side will feel a nice stretch. Hold the position for about 5 counts, then switch over to the other side. Make sure that your body continues to face forward. If you bend forward at the waist you will not feel as much of a stretch. Please maintain normal breathing while you do this exercise.

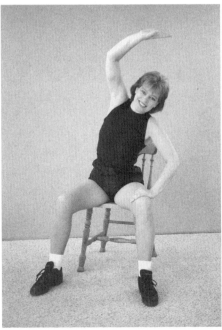

Modified Toe Touch

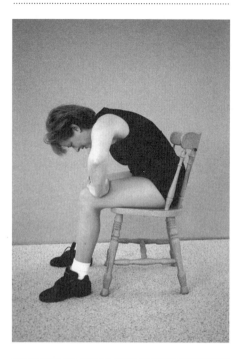

With your feet slightly apart and flat on the floor, put your hands on your knees, wrists outside, and lean forward so your elbows stick out to the side. This is a toe touch without going all the way to the floor. Raise your head to look straight ahead and flatten your back. Make sure your back is not arched, since that position puts strain on your lower back. Now drop your head, roll your shoulders forward, and round your back like a cat. Lift your head and straighten your back again. Flatten, round, flatten, round. After 3 repetitions, roll up to an upright position one vertebra at a time, beginning at the small of the back and rolling up through each vertebra, all the way through the shoulders and the neck.

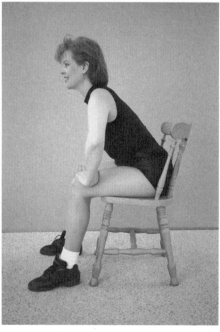

Shoulder Rolls and Lifts

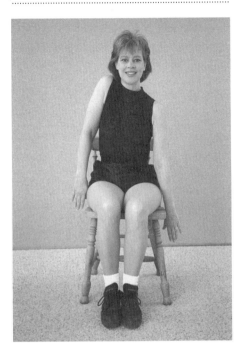

Roll both shoulders back and around. Do this about 4 times, then change directions going forward. Now lift the right shoulder up, hold, and then let it drop. Lift the left shoulder up, hold, and then let it drop. Notice the exercise in the picture.

Hamstring Stretch

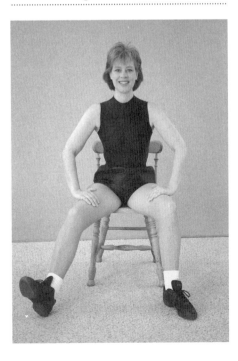

Extend your right leg, then stretch your right toes back. Now do the same with your left leg. Repeat with each leg. The knee does not need to be straight. The stretch is easier with the knee bent if you are sitting in your chair.

Circles

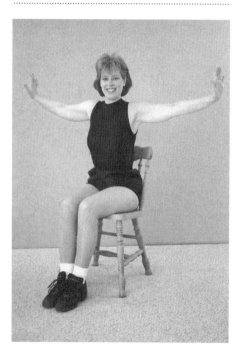

Because later we will do exercises with weights, do not do as many repetitions in these arm exercises. Just loosen up.

Extend both arms out to the side with your hands held up as though you were pushing away the walls. Make small circles forward to a count of 16, then change directions and take 16 counts backward.

Windshield Wipers

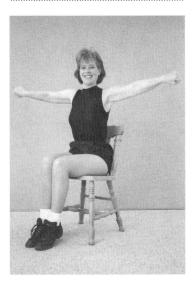

With both arms extended to the side, bend at the elbows, allowing your forearms, wrists, and hands to drop straight down. Then return them to a straight position, just like the windshield wipers on your car. Do this 16 times.

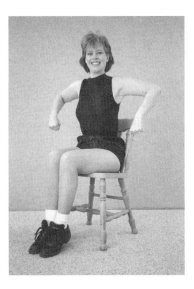

Release Move

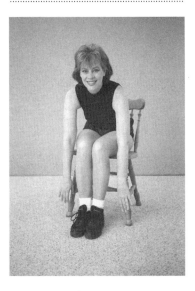

Now do a release move. This is a relaxing movement to prevent your arms from feeling sore. Let your arms drop straight down and shake them out all the way from your shoulders before doing the next arm exercise.

Crisscross

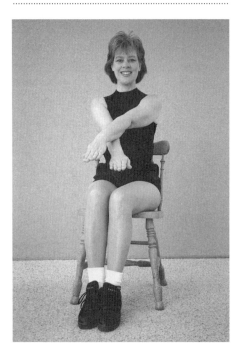

Crisscross your arms and move them up and down in front of you. Go up and down 3 times. Keeping your arms crisscrossed, turn to your right from the waist and move your arms up and down on your right side 3 times. Then repeat this on your left side.

Release Move

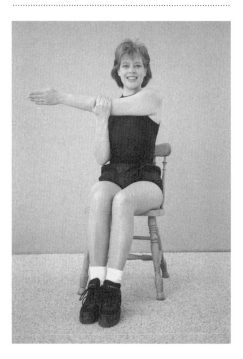

Here is a second release move that relaxes your arms. With your left hand, grab your right elbow and pull your right arm across your body. Repeat this with your left, grabbing your left elbow with your right hand.

Shoulder Swings

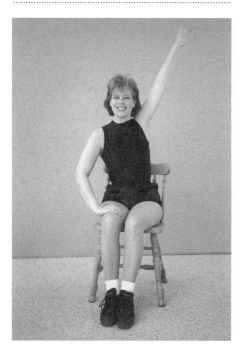

Beginning with the right arm, do 4 giant shoulder swings forward. Move your arm as one unit, gently swinging it like a pendulum from the shoulder and going all the way around in a big circle. Then do 4 giant swings backward. Repeat this with the left arm. Remember not to do this too fast or roughly. You may find one side stronger and more flexible than the other. This is normal.

Side Twists

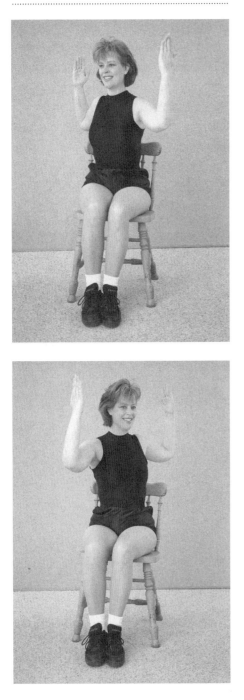

It is important to keep the waist flexible, since this helps our back as well. Plant your feet flat on the floor so they don't shift during this exercise. Now sit a bit forward in your chair to avoid hitting the back as you move. Extend your arms out to the side, then bend your elbows so your hands are facing inward and your fingers are pointing up toward the ceiling. Notice the position of the arms in the photograph. Twist to the right and left from the waist, 16 times each side.

Combination

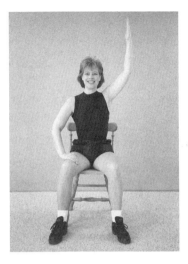

One exercise does not hit all the spots, so this exercise combines three different stretches. Start by stretching your right arm straight up above your head. Now tilt your body to the left, stretching your right side. Your right arm will be directly above your head. Turn your body toward the left, and reach out your right hand as if you were going to push against the wall on your left. Now come back to your normal sitting position and release. Repeat this to the left side. The count should sound like this: stretch, over, turn, sit (release). Do this exercise 4 times on each side, keeping your breathing relaxed and normal.

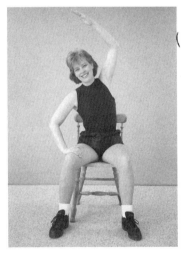

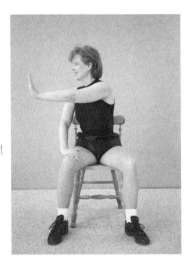

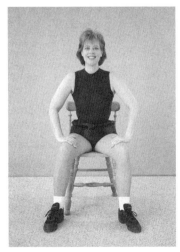

Walk Down the Chair

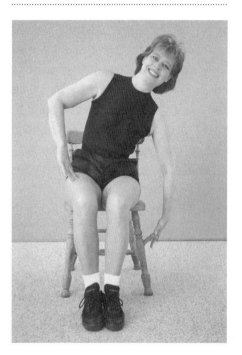

Sitting straight in the chair, let the fingers of your right hand walk down the leg of the chair as far as they will go, for 8 counts. Then walk them up for eight counts. Then the left hand walks down the chair 8 counts and walks up 8 counts. Repeat this once more on each side. It is important that your body remain straight as you walk your fingers down the chair. Line up your torso, shoulders, and head so they all face forward. It is not necessary to walk all the way to the bottom of the chair. It is more important that the body remains straight and doesn't collapse forward.

Wall Pushes

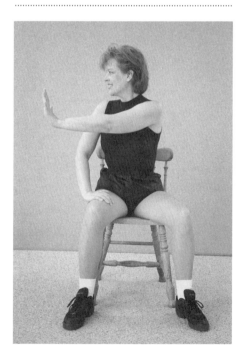

With the wrist flexed and the palm up, extend your right arm across the front of your body, and pretend to push your hand against the wall on your left side. Your body will twist if your feet remain fixed on the floor. Push with your right hand 8 times. Now push with your left hand across your body toward the right wall. Do this 8 times. Repeat 8 counts on each side.

All-Position Stretch

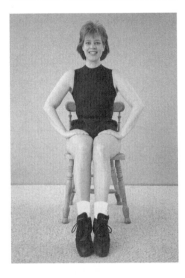

A wonderful ankle stretch that encompasses all the foot stretches begins with your legs extended out in front of you. It is just fine if the knees bend during this exercise. *Point* your toes (both feet at the same time). *Flex* your toes back. *Roll* your toes out to the side (I think of this as "duck feet"). *Push* them down so the toes are pointing at the floor (they are still turned out to the side). *Turn* them back to position one (pointed toes.) Point, flex, roll, push, turn. Repeat this about 5 times, using a continuous movement. It is important to exercise the ankles, so think of this as an important part of your workout.

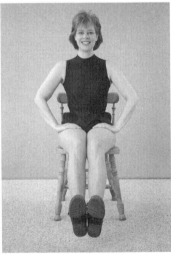

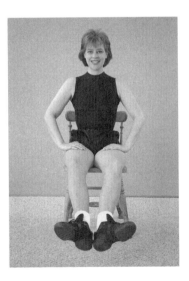

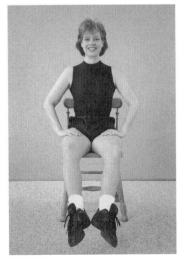

Ankle Circles

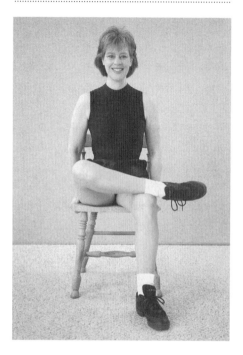

Cross your legs with your right calf over the left knee. This can be a difficult position for some, but try to do it as comfortably as you can. Not only will this exercise help your ankles, it will also make your legs more flexible.

Now circle your ankle first one way, then the other. Now for the tough part. With your ankle still placed on your thigh, lift your lower leg toward your body till your foot is 4–6 inches off the ground. This will push the crossed leg toward your body and create a nice stretch. It will also strengthen your upper leg. Now do the circles and lift/stretch with the other leg. This is an exercise that many struggle with at first but find easier and easier as time goes by.

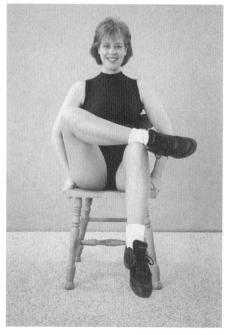

Bent Leg Lifts

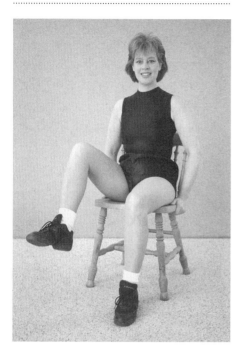

We are going to do a type of leg lift that is a bit unusual, so read carefully. With your legs apart and feet squarely on the ground, pretend that each leg has on it a full cast from upper thigh to ankle. Now lift your right leg up and down 10 times. Imagine the cast is holding your leg in one position, so your knee remains bent at exactly the same angle. Now do 10 lifts with the left leg. If you don't imagine the cast, you will lift using the knee rather than the thigh. As you progress with this exercise, you will notice the difference and feel the thigh muscle doing the work.

Isometric Thigh Closes (The Clam)

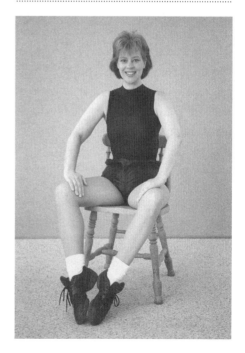

Place your feet together and let your knees separate, like a clam shell that is opening. Now place your hands on the inside of each knee and as you try to close your knees, use your hands to try to keep them apart. Count up to 5. If your knees and your hands are pushing at the same time with the same amount of pressure, your position should not change. Repeat to another count of 5. Later, lengthen the amount of time you do this press.

This exercise can be done anywhere and at any time. It works on the principle of isometrics, or of one force working against another. So not only will the inner thighs be strengthened but also the arms will benefit. Always remember to breathe while doing this isometric exercise.

The stomach is an area many people are concerned about. You probably wonder how you can exercise your stomach while sitting in a chair. Here are a few great exercises that will get your stomach in shape.

Stomach Isometrics

Sit in a relaxed position in the chair with your feet on the floor, making sure your waist or back does not collapse or arch. Count to 10. On each count, pull in and tighten your stomach muscles, then relax them again. When you reach 10, hold in an extra count before releasing. This exercise is great because the muscles in your stomach contract in the same way as they do during a sit-up. You should feel them move in as you tighten them, and release to an expanded position when you relax. As with any exercise, you should exhale while contracting your muscles, and inhale during the release.

This exercise can also be done anywhere. It is great because most people don't pull in their stomach muscles when doing any stomach exercises. It is also amazing to see the stomach muscles working while the rest of the body is relatively still and inactive.

Chair Sit-Ups

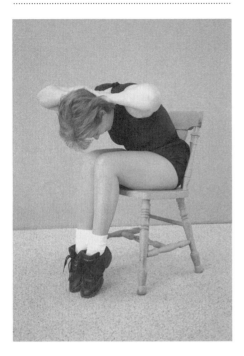

Most people don't like sit-ups because they don't like to get down on the floor. A hard floor can hurt the small of their back, or it may rub on their spine or tailbone. Now you can try your sit-ups in your chair. With your feet together and your hands secured behind your head, bend forward toward your knees, then straighten back up to a sitting position. Begin with 10 sit-ups, and add on 10 more at a time until you feel you have reached your sit-up potential.

Leg Lifts

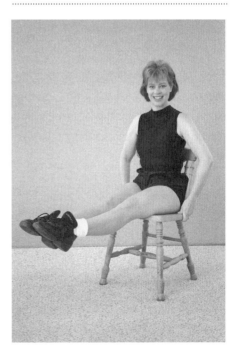

Sit-ups are great stomach exercises, but they focus on only part of our stomach area. Hold on to the side of your chair and extend your legs straight out in front of you. Now slowly lower your legs to about an inch above the floor. Hold. Lift them back up, then lower them again to an inch above the floor. If you do this slowly and hold that stomach muscle as we did in the first stomach isolation, you should feel a nice stomach contraction.

Now for the toughie. Do this again, this time crisscrossing your feet. Hold in that stomach muscle!

■ Aerobics

Because many people feel unsteady or rushed when they do aerobic exercise, most of the aerobic exercises that we will do, including the warm-ups and cool-downs, are done with the support of the chair or wall if need be. If you are comfortable moving without a support, feel free.

Aerobic exercise is often misunderstood. It means that we move our feet and arms at the same time so the lungs and heart work more effectively. The best way to do that is to begin with the legs and add the arms. First we stretch and warm up the legs, then we add some easy arm movements. The arms should move so they come up to heart level. Most people think that unless they work out to a point of breathlessness, they are not doing aerobic exercise. Not so. Aerobics should be done comfortably so that you can talk all through your workout. If you are so breathless that you can't speak, cool it! Tone down your workout. It won't be as effective as a moderate workout.

This aerobic workout is also low impact. That means that we do not jump and jar or put undue stress on the feet, ankles, knees, and legs. It is safe for those who have problem joints—like me.

Hamstring Stretch

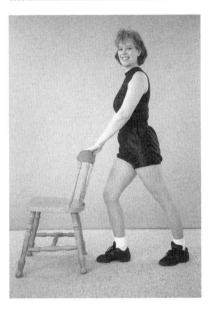

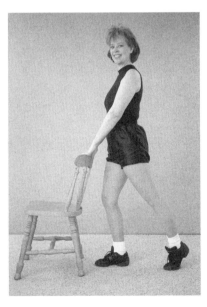

Even if you use a walking or bicycle machine, you should stretch out your hamstrings before starting your aerobic workout. Stand directly behind your chair, holding onto the back with both hands. Extend your left leg behind you until your right knee is somewhat bent. Most of your weight should be on your bent right leg. Now straighten your left leg through the heel, pushing your heel down into the ground. Hold this stretch. Now change, stretching the right leg.

Now return to the left leg, same position. This time lift your back heel up off the ground and then lower it to the ground. Repeat this 5 times, then switch legs.

We are going to include a third exercise in this stretch. Returning to the first leg and position, remember your front leg is bent. Now bend one inch farther into your front leg (or two inches, if you can do it), then return to the original position. Repeat this 5 times. Then do the same exercise with the other leg. This will strengthen your thigh muscles.

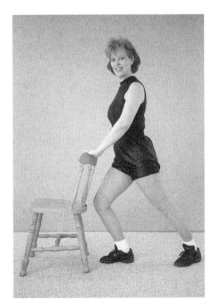

Plié

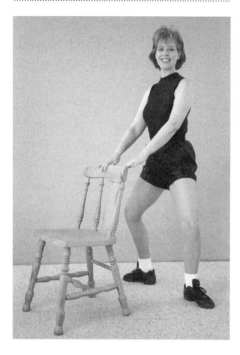

This is an exercise done by dancers to warm up their legs. With your feet a little more than shoulder width apart, your toes turned out slightly, and your upper body straight, bend into your knees so your knees go out over your feet. Return to straight legs. Do this 5 times.

Now do your plié, so you begin in a bent-knee position. Bend your knees a little more, so you go down one more inch, then return to the original bent-knee position. Do this 5 times.

Do your plié once again. While your knees are bent, lift your heels up and let them down 5 times.

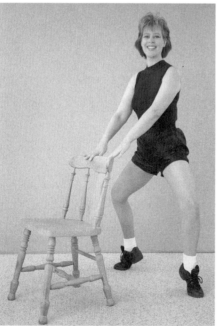

Points and Lifts – 1

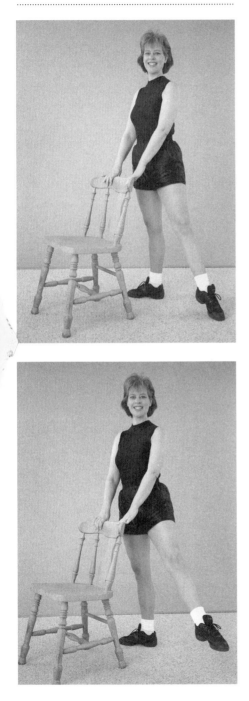

Holding on to the back of your chair, point your right foot out to the side 5 times. Now after you point the foot to the side, lift the leg 5 times (5 points and 5 lifts). When you lift your leg, don't feel you have to lift it high. It is more important that your body is able to stay in a straight upright position. Now do the same thing on the left side.

Points and Lifts — 2

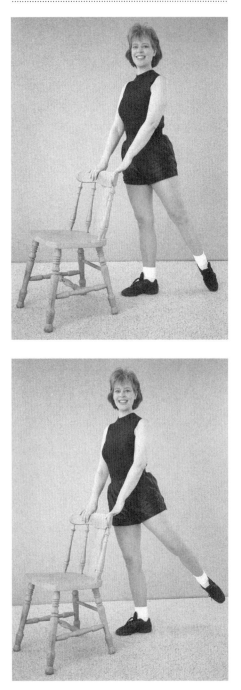

Starting with the right leg, we are now going to do 5 points back. Then 5 lifts back. When lifting the leg backward, don't try to lift very high—only as high as you can without leaning forward. Now switch to the left leg.

Adding Arm Movement – 1

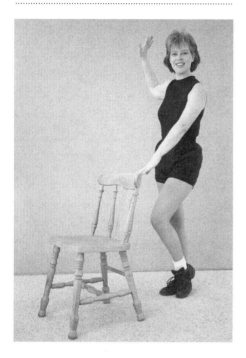

We are going to make some easy movements with the feet and, more importantly, add some arm swings. If you feel at all unsteady, please just swing one arm at a time while holding on to the back of the chair with your other hand.

Feet: Step to the right side, tap the left foot next to the right. Step to the left side, tap the right foot next to the left. Repeat.

Arms: We want your arm to move above your heart. So you may swing the arm under and up, or over like you are waving to a friend across the yard.

Adding Arm Movement – 2

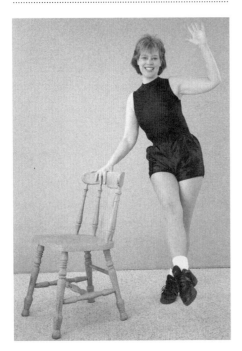

Now let's try a variation.

Feet: Step on your right foot, and let your left foot kick across your body. Now step on your left foot, and kick your right foot across your body. If you kick your legs across and not straight ahead, you won't kick your chair! It also makes you feel like you are on Broadway. Repeat and add the arms.

Arms: Each time you kick with your foot, give the arm a nice high wave. You may wave the same arm if you don't want to let go of the chair, or you may alternate arms each time you kick.

Both exercises should be done for about 5 minutes, so you get your arms and legs going nicely. The one complaint most people voice about aerobic exercise is that it is repetitious and boring. I agree. It is also difficult to do lots of different movements one after another. So if you have favorite movements that include arms and feet moving together, by all means do them. If you can Charleston or twist or do the funky chicken—go for it! Those are all great aerobic exercises. Do something that you like and that feels comfortable.

Walking

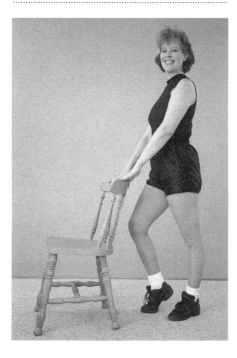

I told you in the introduction that we do walking in our program. Now is the time to do your walking. Here are some suggestions for where and how to walk.

1. You can walk in place, standing behind your chair and holding on to the back. This is a little like a walking machine—it gives you support, and you don't need a lot of room to do it.

2. You can walk around your house, moving from room to room or in any pattern that works with the layout of your home.

3. You can walk around the outside of your house, or walk around your yard.

4. You can walk around your block.

5. If you have a park or walking path near, you can walk there.

6. You can walk your dog. Or your goldfish or your cat, if you choose.

7. You can walk up and down your stairs. If you live in a place that has concrete stairs, please note that the hard surface may not be comfortable or ideal for walking or climbing. It may cause your feet, legs, or joints to feel sore.

8. You can carry weights to enhance your walk. If you do, I recommend that you swing your arms so the weights come up to heart level.

9. You may postpone your walk to earlier or later in the day. You don't have to do it now. Some people prefer to drive to a mall and walk at a different time of day. Or drive later (or earlier) to a park or walkway for their walk. Great! Just be sure to do your warm-up and cool-down then.

After walking, I like to do my cool-down against a wall. You may use the back of your chair instead, if you prefer. One exercise below is difficult to do without the benefit of a wall. I will let you know which one it is when you get to it. You may choose to move to a wall at that time, or simply postpone that exercise until later.

Hamstring Stretch

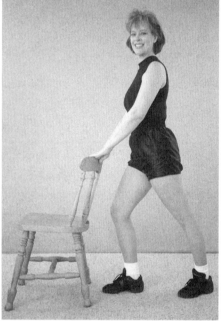

Pressing against the wall (or holding the back of your chair) put one foot out behind you and press your heel into the floor. Your front leg is bent and is supporting the majority of your weight. Now change legs and press the other heel into the floor. Hold your heel down for a count of 8. You may recognize this exercise from our warm-up. We are now using it to cool down and stretch the back of the hamstring.

Bottom Kicks

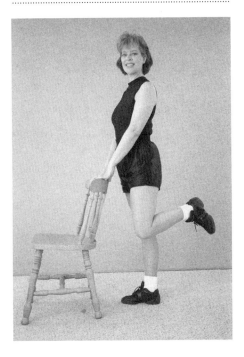

Support yourself against the wall or hold the back of the chair with both hands and, with your right or left leg, try to kick your bottom. You won't ever kick your bottom, but try anyway. Do 10 kicks with the one leg, then 10 kicks with the other.

Back Leg Lifts

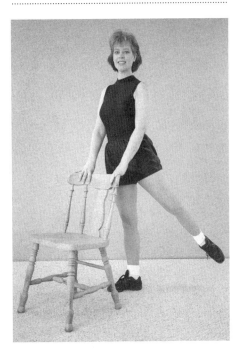

Lean against the wall or hold on to the back of the chair with both hands, and lift your right leg back from the hip 10 times. Remember it is more important to lift your leg without letting your body lean forward than it is to kick very high. Now repeat this 10 times with the left leg.

Bottom Holds

We have been trying to come up with a good name for this exercise, but "Bottom Holds" seems to describe it best. This is an isometric exercise that you can do anywhere—except when you are sitting down, which is why it comes in here during the wall exercises. Count to 10. On each number, tighten your bottom muscles, then relax them. On 10, really squeeze your muscles. This is a great exercise to do while you are waiting in line at the supermarket or the post office.

Grow Two Inches

Many of us have poor to middling posture. As we grow older, we realize the importance of having good posture. It helps us maintain a strong, straight skeletal frame and guards against the stooping and other effects that commonly occur with osteoporosis.

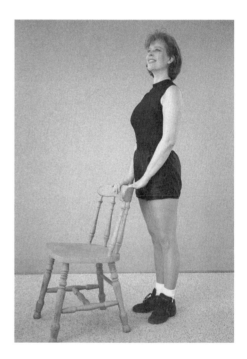

In this exercise—another great one for when you are standing in lines—you imagine that you have a string pulling you up through the top of your head. On the count of 1, feel as if you have grown two inches taller, stretching all the way from your heels to the crown of your head. Feel that string pulling you up to your full height, then relax. Repeat this on the counts of 2, 3, 4, and 5.

One day as my class was doing this exercise, I noticed a woman standing on her tiptoes on each number, then lowering herself to flat feet on the relaxation. However, this exercise isn't intended for the legs and feet, as this woman thought, but for the center of your body around your hips and rib cage, chest, and head/neck area. Feel the string pull you up through your middle, pulling your rib cage up and open.

Wall Push-Ups

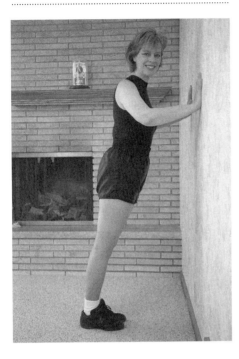

(This is it! This is the one that is difficult to do without a wall.)

This is a favorite exercise because it is difficult to find exercises that strengthen the chest and arm area that are not floor exercises. If you stand about a foot away from the wall with your feet together and your hands about shoulder-width apart on the wall at chest level, you will be able to do push-ups. Be careful not to place your hands too high, at head level, or too low at waist height. I like to place my palms on the wall, but others prefer their knuckles. If you do choose the knuckle method, please remove all rings first.

Keeping your body straight, lower it toward the wall. Bend from the ankle and stop just before you reach the wall. Now push back. Start with 10 push-ups. When you feel comfortable with that number, do 20, 30, or 40. Rest and shake out your shoulders and arms after each set of 10. Several of my students like to do their push-ups on their knuckles, and others clap between pushes just as if they were doing them on the floor.

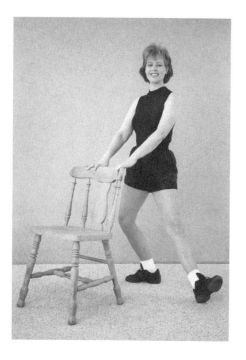

At this point we will be returning to our chairs for the weights section. If you have walked for a long time and would like a few more exercises for stretching out and cooling down, let me make some suggestions. Repeat the section we did in warm-ups with the Plié exercises. Those are the exercises that have the feet apart and flexing into the knees. See page 26. We also did an excellent Hamstring Stretch at the very beginning of our exercises (on page 25), and you may do it here with the aid of the wall or the back of your chair. Extend your right leg out to the side. Your left leg is bent and is supporting the majority of your weight, while your right leg is straight. Now pull your toe back toward you. Repeat this exercise on the left side.

■ Weights

Before beginning the weights exercise, there are a few things to review or consider. First, sit in your chair as if you were going for a haircut. Most hair stylists will tell you to keep your feet together and flat on the floor; otherwise you will be sitting crooked. The same is true for your weight exercises. Sit tall, with your feet flat on the floor. Each exercise will have two sets of numbers, the *repetitions* and the *sets*. A *repetition* is the number of times you will do each exercise at one time. A *set* is the number of groups of repetitions that you will do, resting between each group for about half a minute. A normal repetition is 8, 10, or 12 times, and so forth. We will begin by doing each exercise twice (2 sets). You can increase your repetitions as you become more confident with each exercise. You may also increase the number of sets you do as you develop muscle tone and strength.

Some people may be concerned that they will become "muscle bound"—maybe start looking like Mr. Universe. Please don't worry about that. Our weights are so light that you don't have to worry about them making you look too muscular.

This is one area that many forget to exercise. Have fun. You will enjoy the strength and tone that these exercises will give your arms and upper body. Each exercise, like our other exercises, is designed to develop several different muscles. So feel the unique benefits of each exercise, paying special attention to the muscles used.

Curls

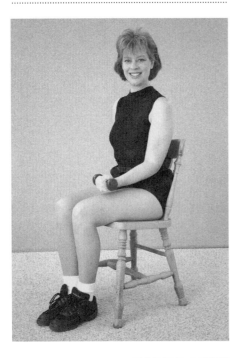

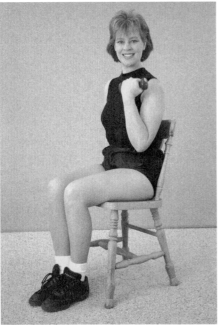

With your feet securely on the ground, hold one weight in your right hand. Press your upper arm (elbow to shoulder) into your torso for support. The upper arm will feel secure and will remain still for the entire exercise. Keep your wrist straight throughout the exercise, and start by holding the weight just above your right knee. Now lift the weight until it *almost* touches your shoulder. Then, with your wrist straight, lower the weight back down to its position above the knee. Repeat this exercise 8 times (repetitions). After a short break, resting the weight upon your knee, repeat the 8 repetitions (a second *set*). Now do 2 sets with the left arm. You may increase your repetitions and sets as you go along, but don't increase them too quickly. Remember, this is only the first exercise. You may very well feel fresh and ready to go at this point, but after a few more exercises you may regret being anxious to increase your numbers too soon.

Windshield Wipers

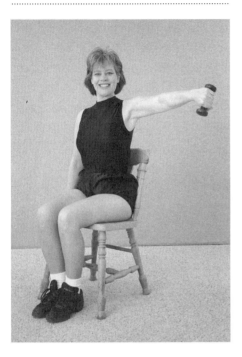

We did this exercise when we began our workout for the arms. It is somewhat more difficult to do with weights, which is why we do it right away in the beginning. With your right arm extended straight out from the shoulder to the side, hold the weight with the back of your hand facing forward. Keeping your shoulder, upper arm, and elbow in place, let your lower arm, wrist, and hand swing down and then back up like a windshield wiper. Do 2 sets of 8 with the right arm, and 2 sets of 8 with the left arm. If you find the exercises too strenuous right away, do 1 set with the right, then 1 set with the left, then go back and repeat 1 set of each.

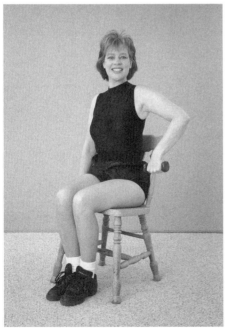

Weed Puller

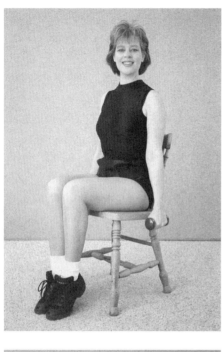

Hold the weight in your right hand, letting your right arm hang straight down at your side. Now lift your right elbow back until your upper arm forms a flat tabletop behind you. I call this the "weed puller," because it is the motion you use to pull out a weed in your garden. Do 2 sets of 8, then repeat the same number with the left arm.

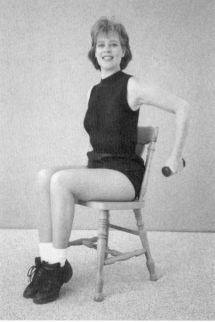

Magnetic Pectoral Pulls

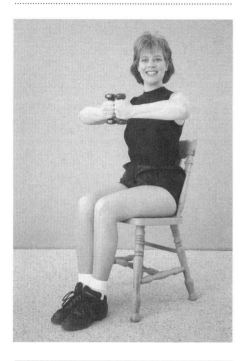

With your elbows out to the side and chest high, hold the weights together in front of your face. Now pull the weights apart, imagining they are magnets trying to connect again, until your elbows can go no farther without going behind you. Then return to your beginning position. Do this exercise in 2 sets of 8 pulls.

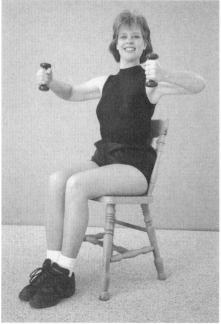

Kissing Weights

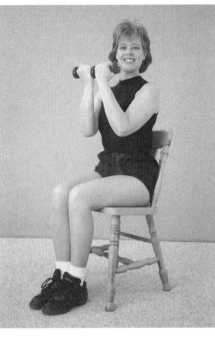

Holding weights in both hands, place them in a "kissing" position in front of your face. Your forearms are touching, as are your pinkie fingers. Pull the weights apart (a little more than shoulder width) and bring them back together again. Do this 8 times. Then repeat for another set of 8.

Release Moves

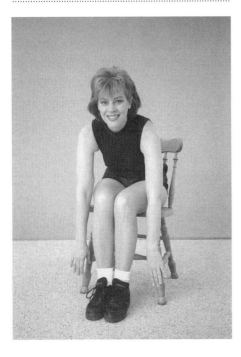

At least two times during your weight exercises, do a release move. This is a way to relax and stretch out your arms and shoulders. I have listed three moves that you can use—and don't use your weights when doing the release moves!

1. Simply let your arms dangle down, with your knees between your arms (see photo), and shake out your arms. At the same time, lift and lower your shoulders. Try doing both shoulders at the same time or each shoulder separately.

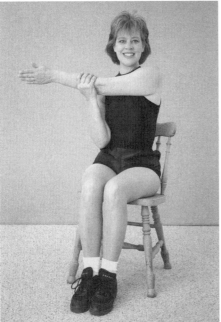

2. Lift your right arm directly up in front of you until it gets to about shoulder level. Grab your elbow with your left hand and pull your right arm across your body, allowing it to stretch out. Repeat with your left arm.

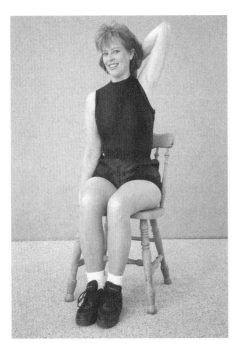

3. Raise your right arm straight up above your head. Now drop your right hand, keeping your elbow still up in the air, and pat yourself on your back. Do the same with your left arm, and pat yourself on your back. Repeat this 2 times on each side.

Waist Stretches

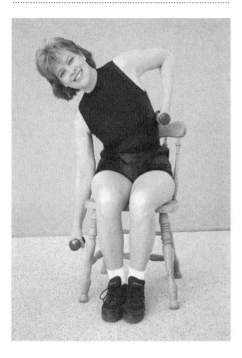

Holding your weights, one in each hand, let your right arm drop to your right side. Your left weight and hand should rest on your left hip. This adds weight for your right arm to lift and lower. Lean to your right side while continuing to face forward, and lower your right arm and weight toward the ground (and the side of your chair). Now lift the right arm and weight up. Go up and down on the right side 8 times. Switch to your left side. Let your left arm and weight lower to your left side. Your right weight should sit on your right hip. Lower and lift the left weight. If you stretch directly to the side without allowing your body to lean forward, you will feel a nice stretch in your side and waist.

Side and Forward Lifts

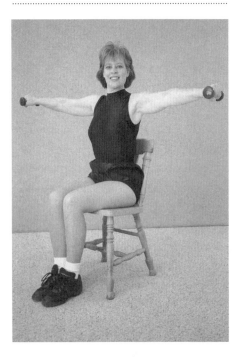

You may do this using only one weight at a time or both. I will explain the exercise as if you are doing both at the same time. Starting with your arms and weights straight down at your sides, lift your arms out to the side, keeping your elbows straight, until they reach shoulder level. Now lower. Do this lift and lower 8 times. Now do the same movement, but raising your arms in *front* of you until they reach shoulder level. Do this 8 times. Repeat 1 more set each of the side and forward lifts.

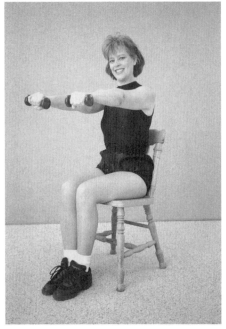

Triceps Lift

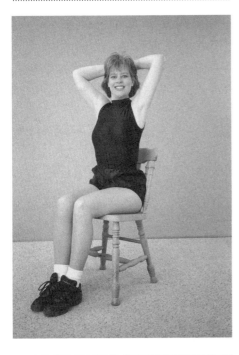

The first thing I always say when we begin this exercise is, "Be careful not to hit yourself in the head with your weights." No one ever has, but I have visions of someone becoming overconfident and hurting themselves during this exercise because it is fun and feels wonderful.

Holding one or both weights with *both* hands, lower your weights behind your head and neck. Now lift and lower your weight(s) from behind your head. Do 2 sets of 8. This is one of the first exercises you will want to do more repetitions or sets of—it feels great and develops a very necessary muscle in your arm.

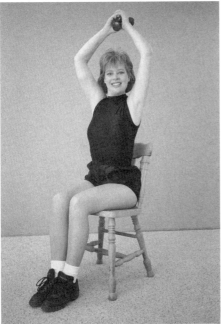

Wrist and Forearm Twists

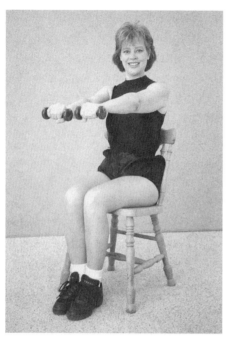

With both arms (and weights) straight out in front of your body, turn your arms so your wrists first face up, then down. Do 2 sets of 8 counts each of these twists.

Final Punches

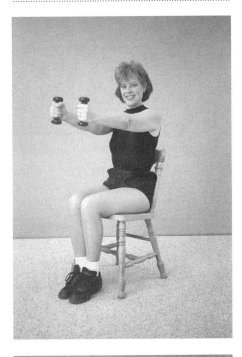

Most people are excited to finally reach this exercise. Using both arms, punch your weights forward and back, then punch them up above your head and down. This is a combination exercise that you should try to do 8 times, rest briefly and then repeat another 8 times.

After this final exercise, place your weights under your chair and do one or two of the release moves (pages 43 and 44) to relax your arms and shoulders.

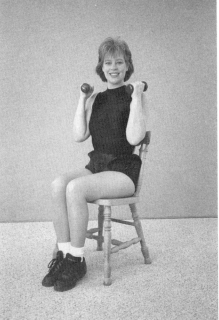

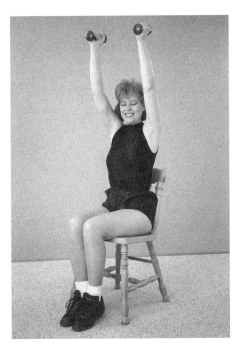

■ Cool-Down

Back Stretch

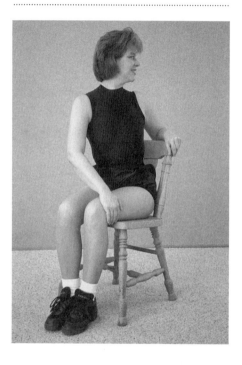

With your feet flat on the floor and your legs and hips facing forward, rest your right arm on the back of your chair and twist and stretch around to your right side. When I do this, my left hand usually finds a comfortable resting spot on my right knee. Hold the stretch, then repeat this to your left side.

Head Stretches

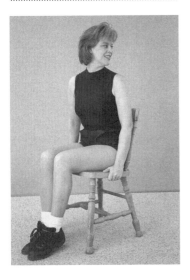

The neck and head are especially delicate, so exercise them slowly and loosely. Some may find it helpful to do these stretches at the beginning of their workout as well as at the end.

1. Look over your left shoulder. Keeping your head level, turn to look over your right shoulder. Repeat 2 times to each side.

2. Start by resting your chin on your chest, then slowly let your head go back until you are looking at the ceiling. Lower to your chin. Repeat.

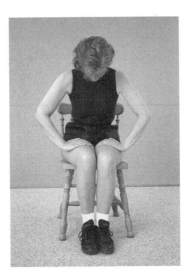

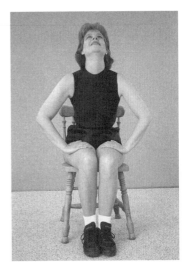

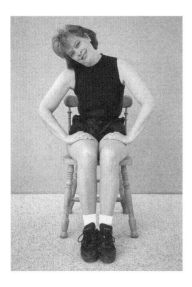

3. Lower your chin to your chest, then let your head swing up until it rests on an imaginary pillow on your right shoulder. Now swing your head back down and up to an imaginary pillow on your left shoulder. Repeat.

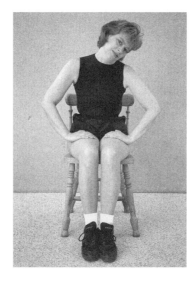

4. Starting with your head erect, first lower it gently, laying your head toward your left shoulder, then let it "flop" (gently of course) over to your right shoulder. "Flop" back to the left shoulder, then back again to the right shoulder. Do this 2 times on each side.

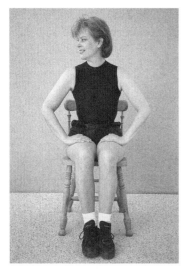

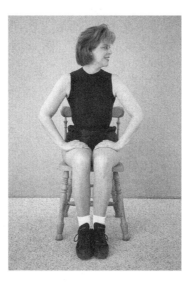

5. Let your head shake gently back and forth in a "no, no" motion.

Face Relaxation

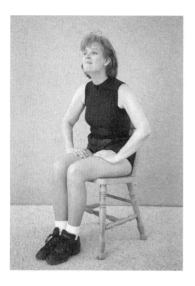

My classes love this section. We do exercises that relax our faces—and make us laugh at the same time. The faces we see on one another are humorous and fun.

1. First, stick out your chin. Bring it back, then jut it out again. Repeat this as many times as you like!

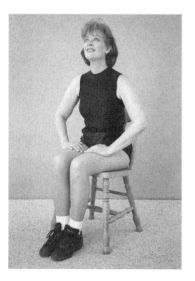

2. Lift your eyebrows toward the ceiling without moving any other part of your face. Repeat this as often as you like.

3. Give a big, big smile (showing teeth, please), then pucker up for a kiss. Do this smile, pucker, smile, pucker about 3 times.

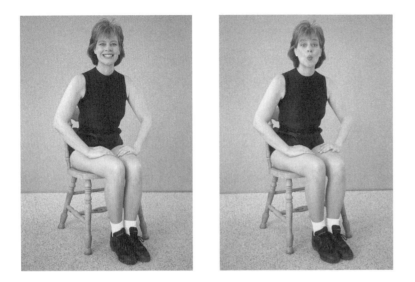

4. Big Mouth. Open your mouth really wide and show your teeth. Repeat this several times.

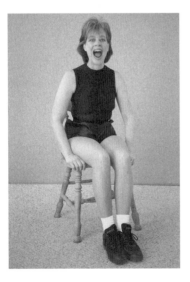

Deep Breathing

We do two exercises in the deep breathing category. The first is an inhaling and exhaling exercise, and we usually do this both in the beginning and at the end of our workout. Begin with your arms hanging in a relaxed position at your sides. Stretch your arms above your head and inhale, as we did in the very first exercise, hold for a few counts, then exhale while lowering your arms. In the course of the program we try to complete at least 6 big inhales/exhales like this. Remember, this helps circulation and improves the lungs and heart.

Our second breathing exercise is one you may need to work up to. We begin by taking in air for 7 counts. Then we hold our breath for a count of 20. The hardest part is the exhaling. Instead of letting all your air out immediately, let it out slowly to a count of 14. We do this exercise at least twice in order to increase our lung capacity and our ability to control our breath. This takes some practice, but it feels really good once it comes easily.

Total Relaxation

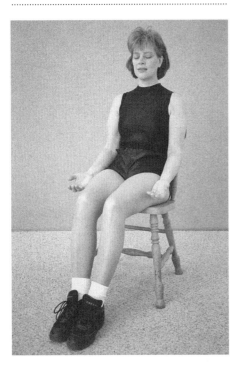

The final stage of our workout is total relaxation, a real favorite. Afterward, you may not feel as if you've exercised at all because you are so relaxed.

Find the most comfortable position you can in your chair, and begin by closing your eyes. Now, starting with your toes and slowly moving upward, focus on one part of your body at a time. As you focus on a particular muscle or body part (for example your heels, shins, stomach, arms, eyes, etc.) concentrate on allowing that part to feel very heavy and totally relaxed. Breathe in and out rhythmically and comfortably as you move from toes to nose to the top of your head.

It may be important during this time to avoid outside distractions and noises that make it hard to concentrate. When you feel totally relaxed and ready, open your eyes and come back to the real world. Take your time, take it slow and easy, don't move immediately or too fast. There's no hurry. You've completed your workout. It's over. You are done. And it feels so good!

Chapter 2

....

Workouts for Problem Areas and Special Conditions

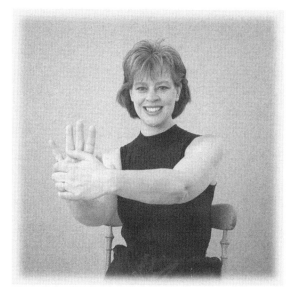

We all have areas that we deem "problem" areas. I enjoy leg exercises because I am flexible, but stomach exercises are harder for me. Therefore, I tend to do more of the stuff I enjoy—the leg exercises—and shy away from those for the stomach. That is probably why my stomach is my problem area.

All of us could use a little pep talk when it comes to emphasizing exercises that deal with our problem areas. So here is my philosophy: Start with the things you don't enjoy or that are harder for you. Then you can look forward to doing the easier more enjoyable things at the end when you may have a little less energy.

But what if your problem areas are not just areas that are a little bit harder? What if you have genuine physical problems and experience pain when doing certain exercises? First, see a doctor. Ask if he or she recommends that you exercise those painful areas. Find out the reason for your stiffness or pain. These may be areas you want to avoid altogether.

Second, if your doctor gives you the okay to exercise, move slowly. When we begin gradually, we are able to build up to greater strength and more comfort easily, if we take our time.

Don't give in to impatience or the need to push until you feel you have the ability to do so safely. We can all be very tuned in to our bodies if we just listen.

What are the most common problem areas, and what can we do about them? In my experience these are the areas that need special attention and care for most of us:

- Back

- Head and Neck

- Upper Legs; Leg Cramps

- Stomach

I have also included information on two conditions that affect us more as we get older:

- Arthritis

- Osteoporosis

■ Back

Many people have back pain, ranging from mild, nagging aches to severe, intense pain. I feel fortunate that I have never had a problem with my back, because I have seen how terribly painful such problems can be. If you have a back problem that requires surgery, by all means follow your doctor's recommendations for treatment.

Many back problems are caused by sitting in one position too long. This can be relieved with some exercise. Remember that exercising once or twice cannot help much, but a consistent and steady plan of exercise can help to relieve many back problems.

Other back problems are due to incorrect posture or position. I remind everyone when doing certain exercises such as sit-ups and back-flexing exercises to avoid going into a swaybacked position. This is when the small of the back is arched so that your behind sticks out. Our body is not designed for this alignment and it puts undue strain on the back. One way to avoid this is to concentrate on proper posture. The exercise where we Grow Two Inches is great for body alignment. The Modified Toe Touch with the hands supporting the body on the knees is also good for the back. In this exercise we allow the back to round, then we straighten it. Notice I said "straighten." That means flattening the back, not arching it.

EXERCISES TO EMPHASIZE

- Grow Two Inches — page 34
- Modified Toe Touch — page 10

■ Head and Neck

Why do I include head and neck in problem areas? The neck is a very small and delicate structure that connects a very large mass (our body) to a very important mass (our head). Because of this we tend to hold it quite rigidly, and as a result often develop stiff necks. So it is important that we relax and strengthen our necks, and we can do this by paying particular attention to the neck exercises during the cool-down. If you do the exercises slowly and carefully, you will feel how soothing it is to stretch out the neck.

EXERCISES TO EMPHASIZE

- Head stretches / cool down — pages 51–52

Face exercises also help us to relax. The face is an area that many people never exercise. When I added face exercises to my program, people loved them. They are a great way to release tension, which really shows on our faces, doesn't it? So smile and pucker up more. It can do more for you than a face-lift.

EXERCISES TO EMPHASIZE

- Face relaxation exercises — pages 53–54

■ Upper Legs

The upper legs may seem like an unlikely problem area as well, but many people have asked me to help them with this. Our upper legs contain some of our body's largest muscles. So if we begin to feel weak in this area, it affects everything—our ability to stand, lift, use our knees, and control our balance.

The seated Bent Leg Lifts shown on page 21 are wonderful for building strength. Begin with fewer lifts, but work up to more and more.

The Aerobics section with the Points and Lifts beginning on page 27, the Walking (shown on page 31) and the Kicks Across are also very good. Many of the exercises listed have an additional part for working the upper leg. You might try the one-inch-lower extension of the Plié (page 26). Or the standing Hamstring Stretch with its one-inch-lower exercise found on page 25. It may seem easy when you look at the exercise, but once you try it, you'll notice how difficult it actually is. Also the Ankle Circles contain an additional exercise that helps to strengthen the thigh. Try lifting the supporting leg when the ankle is resting in cross-legged position (page 20). If you have a problem with this area, do not shy away from doing more repetitions. It will certainly give you more strength. Remember the saying, "Use it, or lose it!" This certainly applies to muscle tone. If you don't exercise certain muscles, you'll lose the strength and tone as well as the flexibility.

EXERCISES TO EMPHASIZE

- Bent Leg Lifts — page 21
- Points and Lifts — pages 27–28
- One-inch lower extension of the Plié — page 26
- One-inch lower extension of the Standing Hamstring Stretch — page 25
- Ankle Circles with Supporting Leg Lift — page 20

■ Leg Cramps

Many people who haven't exercised in a long time, or go too fast, get leg cramps. Leg cramps are also very common for pregnant women. Most cramps are not dangerous, though they can indicate a lack of calcium in the diet. If you do get cramps, either when exercising or later at home or at night in bed, try the exercise that we do to warm up called the Hamstring Stretch. When you are standing or sitting, simply pull your toe back toward your body and hold that position. This will help relieve a leg cramp, and it will also help you avoid leg cramps in the future. When I am lying in bed I frequently flex my foot a few times to help prevent cramping. You may even want take hold of your foot with your hand and pull the toe back if you feel the need for a greater stretch.

EXERCISES TO EMPHASIZE

- Hamstring Stretch — page 25

Stomach

As I mentioned earlier, the stomach is my problem area. I will share only a few thoughts to help those of you who are like me. Do a stomach exercise every day. Consistency is very important. The Stomach Isometrics (on page 22) are very good. Tightening the stomach muscles is the key to all the other stomach exercises you can do. Many people tell me, "I exercise all the time. I do all kinds of sit-ups, but nothing helps." The key lies not in doing all kinds of exercises but in doing them correctly. When doing stomach exercises, it is of utmost importance that you tighten your stomach muscle like we do in the Stomach Isometrics, or the exercise won't do you very much good. So practice. Get the feel of tightening that muscle before you try all those other exercises. Do it right, and do it consistently. We all have habits, and stomach isometrics is one of those good habits we can develop. Get yourself into the habit of doing your stomach exercises at the same time every day— while you are brushing your teeth, for example. Try doing a few before you buckle your seat belt, or every morning when you first get up. Then you will have a habit you can be proud of, as well as a strong and flat stomach.

EXERCISES TO EMPHASIZE

- Stomach Isometrics — page 22

■ Arthritis

If you feel a stiffness or pain in your joints, it may be arthritis; one person in seven suffers from arthritis to some degree. Arthritis has many causes and takes many forms in the body. If you suspect you have arthritis, see a doctor for a diagnosis as well as a recommendation before exercising.

The most common arthritis is osteoarthritis, which is the wearing down of the cartilage that cushions our joints. This type of arthritis is more and more common in people as they grow older.

It is important for people who suffer from arthritis to have a good exercise program. Exercise works for our joints the way that oil works to lubricate a car. It increases healing by allowing the fluids to "grease" our joints. Exercise also helps the muscles surrounding an arthritic joint to become stronger and more supportive. So even if you feel some pain, please don't stop exercising. Do, however, choose your exercises and methods carefully.

Remember the three C's of exercise: especially if you have arthritis. Exercise *carefully* by selecting a program that is right for you. Exercise *correctly* and *consistently* to prevent injuring your joints and to build up the muscles that will allow your joints to work more freely.

All the exercises demonstrated in the One-Hour Chair Program in chapter 1 are won-derful for people with arthritis. The chair program is low impact, which means that it does not put undue stress on your ankles, knees, hips, and legs. That is important if you suffer from arthritis.

The chair program also stresses positioning and alignment. It is important that you not put too much stress on any one bone or joint when sitting or standing. Carefully study each photograph as you exercise so that you align your body correctly.

Also be careful where you exercise. Running, walking, or exercising on floors that are hard—made of cement or placed directly on cement—are not great for the joints. If you exercise by climbing stairs, check the hardness of the stairway or you may end up with aching knees and ankles.

Go slowly. Warm up more thoroughly. Do gentle rotations. Do them in a relaxed manner. Take it easy!

For your shoulders, do the Shoulder Rolls and Lifts shown on page 11 as well as the Shoulder Swings on page 15. You may find that one arm or shoulder is more mobile than the other. This is quite common.

If you have stiffness in your elbows, do some of the weight-lifting exercises such as Curls and Final Punches found in the weight section beginning on page 37. You may want to do them without weights. This works the elbows without putting stress on that area.

Ankles will become more flexible with the rotations and pointing and flexing exercises found on pages 19 and 20. These are great to warm up with before doing a more strenuous exercise. The Hamstring Stretches on pages 11 and 25 also stretch out the ankles. Do the Plié on page 26 with the heel lifts. Women who wear high heels really benefit from the ankle exercises shown on pages 19–20. I do them all the time to relieve and prevent ankle and leg stiffness.

EXERCISES TO EMPHASIZE

- Shoulder Rolls and Lifts — page 11
- Shoulder Swings — page 11
- Curls — page 38
- Final Punches — page 49
- All-Position Stretch — page 19
- Hamstring Stretches — pages 11, 25
- Plié with Heel Lifts — page 26

If you have knee problems, as I do, listen to what your doctor tells you—but listen carefully to your body also! My doctor told me to do a weight-lifting program to strengthen the muscles in my upper legs. I found this to be too difficult. So I began gradually by doing exercises with no weights. I did Leg Lifts (page 23), Bottom Kicks (page 33), and bicycling to strengthen my muscles as well as work my knees. I learned my limitations and built up from there. I am careful to do low-impact exercising and to exercise on a floor with a little give to it. When I walk, I try to walk on softer ground rather than on hard cement sidewalks. I allow myself to develop habits that feel good and make sense when it comes to my problem areas.

If you are concerned about your hips, try some Front and Back Leg Swings (page 93). The Points and Lifts (pages 27–28) are also very good for the hips. Be careful to let the hip do the work. By that I mean stand straight with good posture and let the movement come from the hip instead of leaning backward and forward with the movement. Move gently. Build up to a comfortable number of repetitions.

EXERCISES TO EMPHASIZE

- Points and Lifts — pages 27–28

- Bottom Kicks — page 33

- Front and Back Leg Swings — page 93

If you have problems with your wrist joints, I will show you some wonderful exercises. First, just rotating the wrist will help to loosen up the joint. Remember to rotate in both directions. If you take hold of your right hand with your left across the upper palm, you will be able to gently stretch the right hand back toward your wrist. Then grasp the right hand in the left across the back of the hand. Gently press it toward the inside of the wrist. Now repeat this exercise with the left hand. See the demonstration in the pictures below.

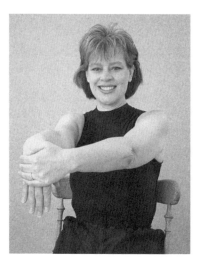
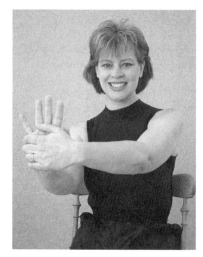

Gently spread your fingers, and stretch each finger by holding it and, with a massage-like motion, stretching the finger from its lower joint nearest the palm. Next work the joints at the knuckle and near the fingernail. Gently working these joints will help lubricate areas that feel stiff. When you do other exercises, such as the arm exercises found on pages 12 through 15, spread your fingers as you exercise. Although you are doing exercises for other areas of your body, this hand position will help your fingers feel wonderful. If you find you have a great deal of pain when exercising, see your doctor immediately.

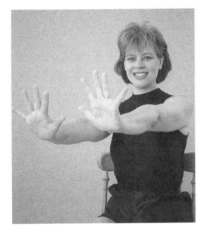
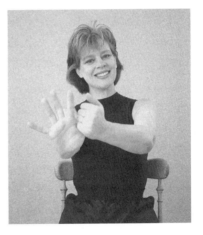

For more on arthritis, check the Additional Reading found at the back of this book. And remember:

- use proper alignment when sitting or standing (or when exercising!)

- do not overdo the weights

- warm up and cool down properly before and after your exercise

- check the area you are exercising on for surface hardness

- select low-impact exercises, and

- exercise consistently (three times a week to improve your condition, twice a week to maintain it).

Your bones, just like your muscles, grow stronger with additional exercise. Don't lose what you have. Improve it instead.

■ Osteoporosis

When your bone mass decreases faster than it is replaced, you have the condition known as osteoporosis. Although this may be caused by a number of things, including poor diet, and may develop in anyone of any age, it is most common in women as they grow older. Some of the most common effects of osteoporosis are the shrinking of the skeletal frame, which affects our posture, and brittle bones. These brittle bones put those with osteoporosis at greater risk for breaks, fractures, and other bone damage.

What can be done? Most physicians recommend exercise. Of course, if you suspect you have this condition, check with a doctor before exercising. Exercise increases the strength of the muscles surrounding the bones as well as the bones themselves. This helps the person with osteoporosis to prevent or reduce some of the common effects.

It is important that those with osteoporosis select a low-impact exercise program, such as the One-Hour Chair Program. It is also important that the program be conducted in a safe area that prevents any risk of falls. Please do your walking section (page 31) with the support of a chair. This will reduce any risk of tripping.

Your posture will improve with the Grow Two Inches exercise found on page 34 as well as by doing the warm-up stretches (page 9) and by using correct body alignment when sitting or standing.

The exercises for building your thigh muscles (pages 20, 21, 26, 27, 28, and 33) will give you greater strength and balance when lowering your body into a chair or trying to stand up from a sitting position. We frequently forget that our thigh muscles help us with movements we take for granted. But when we are concerned about preventing injury to our bones, those movements may give us cause for worry. Again, remember the three C's of exercise: exercise *carefully,* exercise *correctly,* and exercise *consistently.*

EXERCISES TO EMPHASIZE

- Walking exercises — page 31
- Grow Two Inches — page 34
- Warm-up stretches — pages 9 & 11
- Exercises for thigh muscles — pages 20, 21, 26, 27, 28, and 33

Chapter 3

....

But I Don't Have Time . . .
The 5-Day Short Program

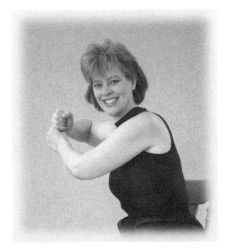

The "But I Don't Have Time..." program is designed for those who are too busy (or too tired) to do the hour-long program described in chapter 1. Remember, I believe that consistency is the key to any exercise program. So, if you only have ten or fifteen minutes each day—or every other day—as long as you are consistent, and persistent, you will get very effective fitness results.

In this chapter, I will recommend a five-day short program for those who have only a few minutes to exercise. Those who can take some time during their lunch hour or break time should find these exercises perfect for that time frame.

Those who find the hour-long program too long or too strenuous should also begin with these shorter workouts. Then you can move on to the longer program at a later time, when you feel ready! You might also consider doing shorter ten-minute exercise sessions twice a day if you would like to build up your endurance.

The exercises in shorter daily programs are all taken or adapted from the One-Hour Program. Most of the daily programs include an exercise from each of the muscle groups, so you will receive a well-rounded program. As I have recommended before, if there is an exercise that you do not feel comfortable with or your doctor recommends avoiding, replace that exercise with another that does feel good and safe to you.

Let's begin!

Warm-Up — Deep Breathing

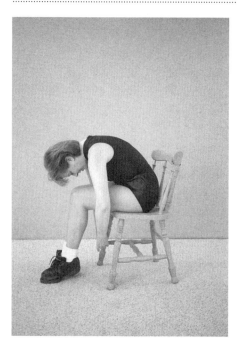

Sitting on the edge of your chair with your feet together and flat on the floor, allow your arms to drop, and exhale and bend forward until your hands are below your knees. Now raise your arms up above your head, inhaling deeply so you feel the air move all the way into your abdomen. Hold the breath, and then exhale, bending forward and letting your arms hang below the knees again. Do this 3 times. Notice the starting and ending positions pictured below.

Shoulder Rolls and Swings

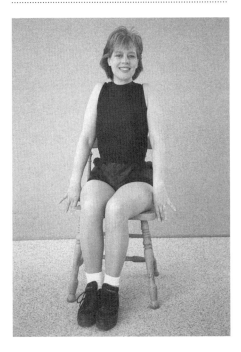

Slowly lift both shoulders up toward your ears, then let them drop. Do this 3 times. Then roll your shoulders forward and around 3 times. Now roll the shoulders back and around 3 times. Next, swing your right arm forward and all the way around in a giant circle. Do this 3 times. Then swing it backward in 3 giant circles. Repeat these giant swings with the left arm, first forward, then backward.

Remember

- 3 shoulder shrugs up and down
- 3 shoulder rolls forward
- 3 shoulder rolls backward
- 3 giant swings forward with the right arm
- 3 giant swings backward with the right arm
- 3 giant swings forward with the left arm
- 3 giant swings backward with the left arm

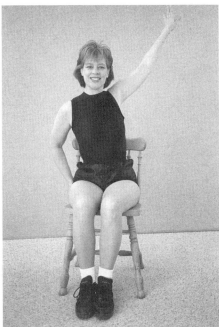

Waist Twists

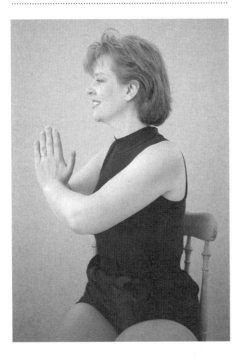

Sitting slightly forward in the chair so you don't hit the back as you move, clap your hands together in front of you at about chest height. Now pull your hands in a bit so your elbows extend out to the side. With your feet remaining in place flat on the floor, twist from side to side 6 times.

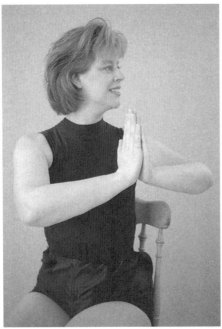

Ankle Stretches

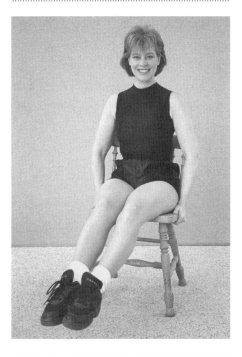

Extending your legs out straight in front of you, point both feet. Then flex both feet back. Do this 5 times. Separate your legs a little and roll both feet outward 5 times. Then roll both feet inward 5 times. If you can do this exercise while sitting on the edge of your chair with your legs just slightly raised off the ground, you can also exercise your stomach. Simply tighten your stomach muscles as you do the exercise, and you will also have completed your stomach workout!

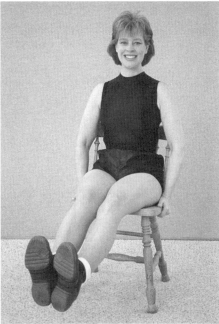

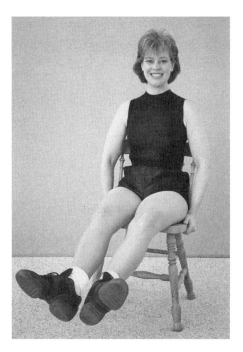

Leg Lifts

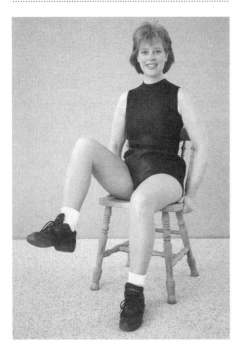

With your legs slightly parted and your feet on the floor, imagine that each leg has a full cast on it from upper thigh to ankle. Lift your right leg 10 times. Now lift your left leg 10 times. The idea of imagining the cast is to lift the leg from your thigh, and not to use or flex your knee.

We will do a combination of two weight-lifting exercises described in the One-Hour Program. When doing these exercises, consider several things. First, our arms are an often-neglected area of our anatomy. Second, these exercises work not only our arms but our upper body as well. Third, weights are not necessary—you can do these exercises without weights if you choose. If you are doing them at work and do not have weights at your desk, pick up something that has a little weight to it and lift that. Please don't lift the copy machine or anything that weighs more than three pounds.

Curls

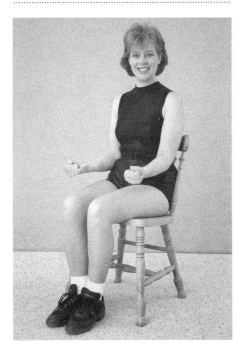

Let's begin with curls. You can do both arms together if you want to cut down on the time needed. With your elbows against your body, hold your hands, with or without weights, just above your knees. Raise your fists up toward your shoulders, hold them for a moment, then slowly lower them to just above the knees again. The slower you do the exercise, the more you work your muscles. Do 8 repetitions on each side (or at the same time).

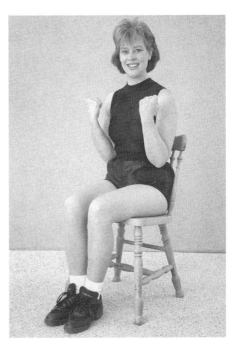

Side Lifts

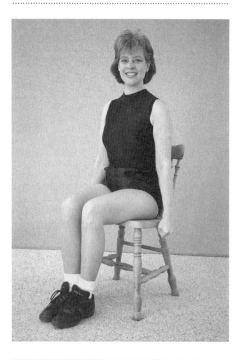

Now, starting with your weights (or just your fists) at your side, lift your arms straight out to the side until they reach shoulder height, then lower. Repeat this 8 times.

Bottom Kicks/Side Leg Lifts

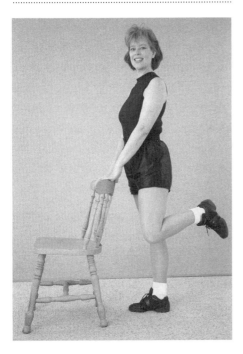

Standing behind your chair, hold on to the back for support. With your right leg, try to kick your bottom. Do this 10 times, then do bottom kicks 10 times with your left leg.

Holding on to the back of your chair, lift your right leg out to the side 10 times. Keep your leg straight and your toe pointed so it creates a nice line from toe to hip, and lift only as high as you can without allowing your body to lean. It may not feel as if you are lifting very high. The height is not important. If you lean with your body, you will not use your leg muscle as much as if you remain upright and lift from the hip. Now lift 10 times to the left side.

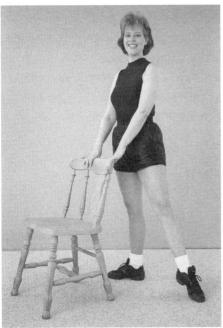

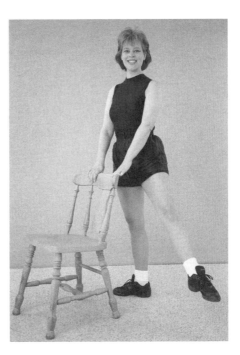

Cool-Down

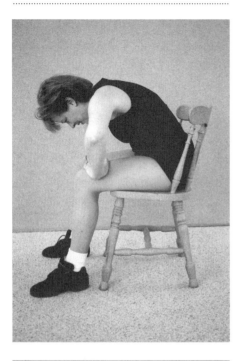

Sit down in your chair. With your knees apart and your feet flat on the floor, place your hands on your knees, wrists outside. Lean forward so your elbows stick out to the side, look straight ahead, and flatten your back. As you support your body weight on your knees, lower your head, roll your shoulders forward and round your back. Now straighten your back again, being careful not to arch it. Round and straighten your back 5 times.

Very gently, roll your head down and around to the right 5 times. Now switch and roll it back the other way.

Now sitting relaxed in your chair, inhale and hold. Exhale slowly. Repeat this 3 to 5 times. You are now finished with the first ten-minute workout. Congratulations!

You may repeat this workout again later in the day if you choose, or go on to the next ten-minute workout tomorrow. Some people choose to exercise every other day. That is perfectly acceptable. Choose times that fit your schedule, and add on more later. Remember, consistency is the key.

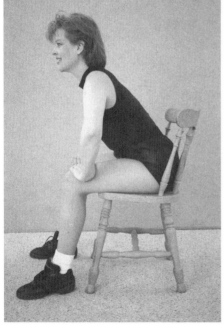

Warm-Up — Overhead Stretch

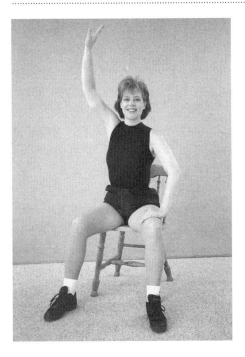

Our warm-up on Day Two will be an overhead stretch. This stretches your arms as well as your torso. Begin with your feet about shoulder width apart and flat on the floor. Now reach up with your right arm, stretching it straight above your head. Turning your palm over as if you were going to wash the ceiling, lean to your left with your hand over your head. You can rest your left hand on your left knee to support part of your weight. Take a nice long stretch, feeling your right side and your arm extending and loosening up.

Now gently try to stretch a little bit more. I call this a pulse. Pulse with your right arm 6 to 8 times, each time trying to reach a little farther.

Repeat this stretch with the left arm. First, focus on a nice long stretch, then do 6 to 8 pulses.

Arms — Little Circles

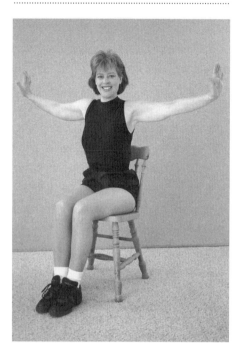

Our arm exercise will be small circle rotations. With your arms extended straight out to the side, hold your palms out as if you were going to push away the walls. Some like to make a drooping fist. This is a perfectly fine alternative. Now rotate the arms forward, making tiny little circles. Begin with 10, then gradually increase to 20 or even 30 as you feel the strength. Shake out your arms. Extending your arms out to the side again, make tiny little circles backward. Begin again with 10, then increase to 20 or 30.

Wall Pushes

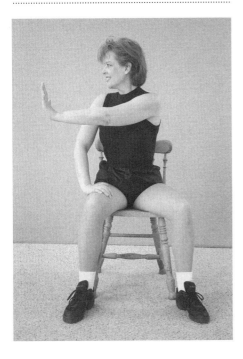

For our waist, we will do wall pushes. With the wrist flexed and the palm up, stretch your right arm across the front of your body as if pushing against the wall on your left side. This stretches your waist, and you should feel a nice twist. Push against the left wall 10 times. Now with the left hand, push across your body toward the right wall 10 times.

Ankle Circles and Lifts

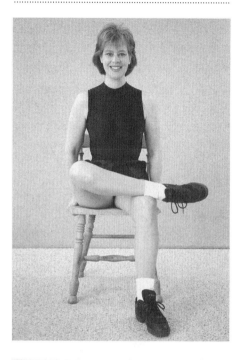

Cross your legs with your right ankle over the left knee. Now rotate your right ankle first in one direction, then in the other. Rotate in each direction about 8 times. It is quite all right to "help" your ankle to rotate by taking hold of your foot with both hands and rotating gently. The purpose of the exercise is to stretch out your ankle, not build up your muscles.

Before moving on to the next exercise, try this variation to strengthen your flexibility and your upper leg. With the right ankle placed on your left thigh, lift your left leg toward your body until your foot is 4–6 inches off the ground. This is a tough exercise for many, but those who have persisted find it feels wonderful. I like to hold on to the edges of my chair while I do these lifts. Begin with 3 lifts and work up to 5.

Repeat the ankle circles with the left ankle. Now try lifting the right supporting leg.

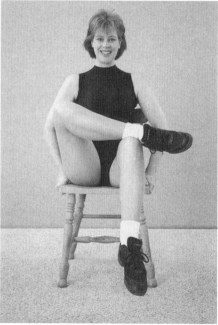

The Clam

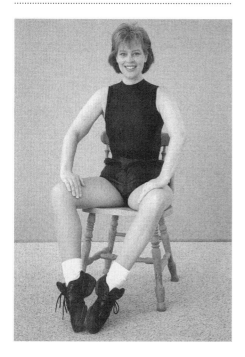

This is an isometric exercise that works not only your upper legs but also your arms. With your feet together on the floor (I try to place the soles of my shoes together), part your knees, like a clamshell that is open. Place your hands on the insides of your inner knees or just above, on your inner thighs. Now try to close your legs while pushing with your hands to keep them apart. The muscles of your legs are pushing against the muscles of your arms. Count up to 8. Take a rest, and try a second set of 8 counts. Over time, you may be able to develop your arms so that your legs never shut.

Chair Sit-Ups

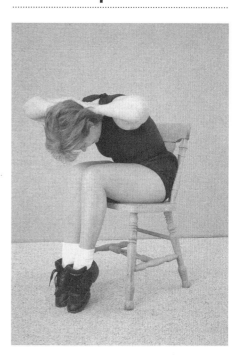

Yes, you can do sit-ups in your chair. Place your legs and feet together. With your hands across your chest or—my favorite—laced behind your head, bend forward toward your knees, then straighten back up to a sitting position. You do not need to touch your knees, but you should be aware of holding in your stomach muscles as you press forward. Begin with 10 sit-ups. If this feels comfortable for you, do one or two more sets of 10 each. I've read that Paul Newman does 200 sit-ups a day. So, in my classes, we joke that our goal is 200. We certainly would love to look as fit as Paul Newman.

Triceps Lift

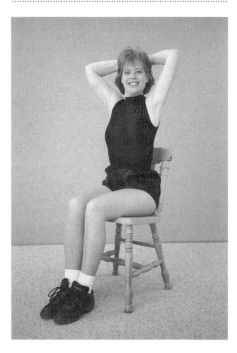

One of the most difficult areas to exercise is the underside of the upper arm, the triceps. It just seems to sag no matter what we do. This is a great exercise for that area. Using your weights—if you choose to and have them handy—hold on to the same weight with both hands and lower it behind your head. Now *carefully* raise and lower the weight behind your head. Do this 8 times. Rest. Then do a second set of 8 repetitions. Increase your sets and repetitions as you feel stronger.

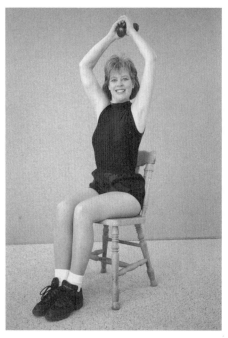

Magnetic Pectoral Pulls

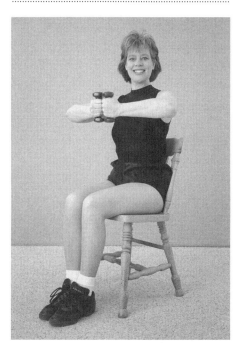

The pectorals are the chest muscles. Many people ignore the upper body when exercising. Others work only the upper body if they emphasize just weight lifting. Working with small weights won't make you look like Mr. Universe, but it will make your feel stronger and healthier.

Hold the weights together in front of you about shoulder height, and lift your elbows out to the sides. Now pull the weights apart, imagining they are magnets trying to connect again. Do 8 pulls, rest, then do 8 more. You may add sets and repetitions as you feel stronger. With the shorter workout, it may take you less time to add to your workout.

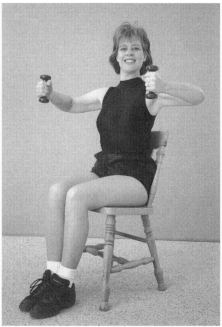

Cool-Down — Shoulder Lifts

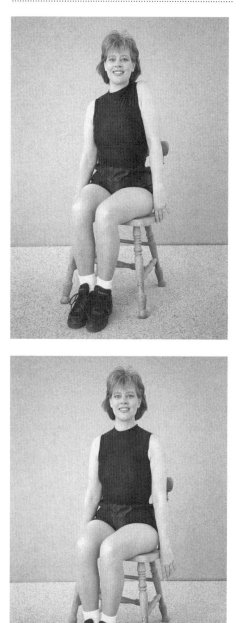

Slowly lift your right shoulder up and lower it 3 times. Now roll it gently forward 3 times, then backward 3 times. Switch to the left shoulder. Do 3 lifts, 3 forward rolls, and 3 back rolls. Do this very slowly, breathing deeply with each lift or roll.

"No, No" Head

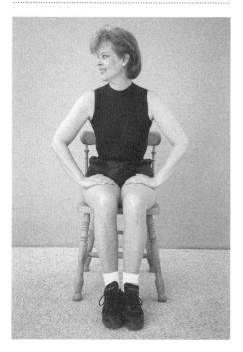

The neck is an area that should be treated with great care. So, very slowly, shake your head to the right and left, as if saying "no, no."

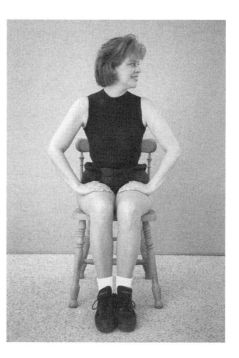

Deep Breathing

Finally, inhale deeply, holding in the air. Feel the breath deep in your abdomen. Now exhale slowly. Take 3 to 5 deep breaths, placing your hands on your stomach to feel your muscles expand and relax. You have completed the second day's workout. Great job!

Today is our walking day. That doesn't mean you need to walk any farther than your own living room or office. See the ideas for walking exercises on page 31, and use your chair if you wish. If you have only 10 minutes to exercise, limit your walking to 3 to 5 minutes.

Grow Two Inches

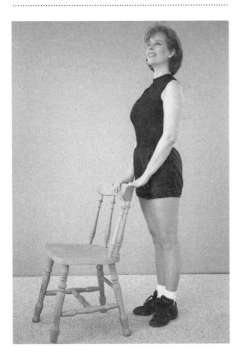

For our warm-up we will grow two inches. Standing behind your chair (you may remain seated if you feel uncomfortable standing) imagine that a string is threaded through your body and comes out the top of your head. Now pull that string straight up and make yourself grow two inches. Then relax. The purpose of this exercise is to feel a nice stretch through your whole body and to improve your posture. You should feel a nice stretch through your hips and rib cage, through your upper body, back, and shoulders. You should also feel your neck and head extend. Do this exercise 5 times, resting after each stretch.

Hamstring Stretch

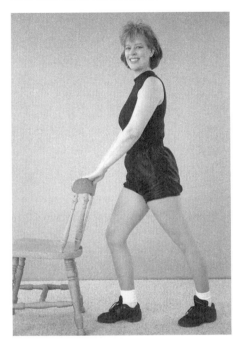

Holding on to the back of your chair with both hands, extend one leg behind. The back leg should be straight, with the front leg bent and supporting most of your weight. Now push your left heel down into the ground, straightening and stretching the back of your leg. Hold this position and feel the stretch. Repeat 8 times.

To exercise your thigh muscle, hold the original position—your back leg straight with the heel pressed into the floor and the front leg bent and supporting most of your weight. Now bend into the front leg one inch more. Come back to the original position, then bend into the front leg one inch more again. Do this bend 5 times.

Repeat all three exercises with the other leg.

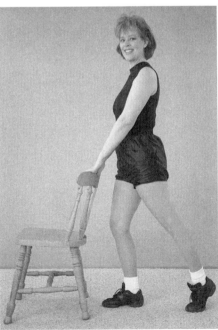

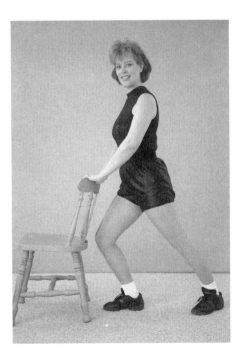

Points and Lifts

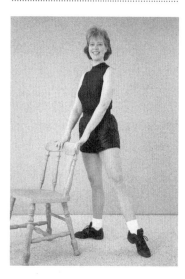

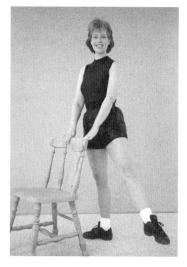

Standing behind your chair with both hands on to the back, point your right foot out to the side (point), then bring it back to the left foot (close). This part of the exercise is for the ankles. Point and close the right foot 5 times.

Now point the right foot, close to the left, then lift the right leg to the side. Repeat this 5 times. The leg need not lift very high. The point of the exercise is to work the hip and upper leg, so try to lift the leg only as high as you can while your body remains upright.

Repeat both the points and the point with lift with the left leg.

Now do the same exercises, but pointing and lifting back. Right leg 5 points back, then 5 points with back lift. Switch legs and do 5 points back with the left foot, then 5 points and back lifts with the left leg.

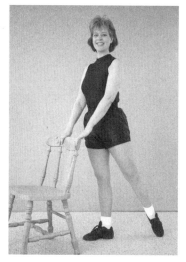

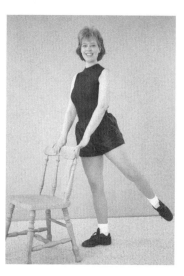

Front and Back Leg Swings

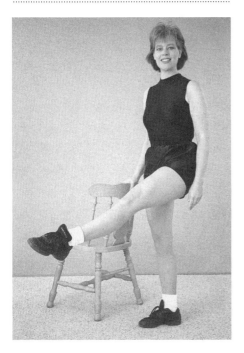

Supporting yourself with your left hand on the chair and your body turned so your left side is closest to the chair, let your outside leg (right) swing back and forth. The leg should be as straight as possible, swinging smoothly, like a pendulum. Swing forward and back 5 times, keeping your body straight. You should feel the movement come from the hip. Some people find their leg bending at the knee as they swing the leg. That is fine as long as the body doesn't begin to sway with the leg. Now repeat with the other leg, turning so your right hand holds the chair.

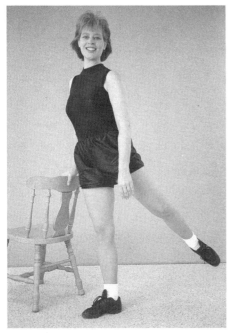

Pliés

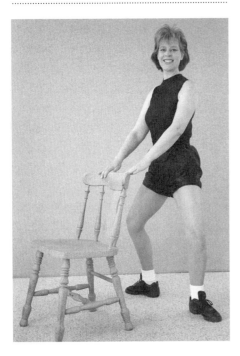

Facing the chair and placing both hands on the back, place your feet about shoulder width apart, turning your toes out slightly. Keeping your back straight and your hips underneath your upper body, lower yourself into your knees. This is called a plié. Your knees should go out over your toes. Plié slowly 5 times. This strengthens your upper legs and improves the flexibility of your knees.

Now start in the plié position with the knees bent over the feet. Lift both heels off the floor. Lift and lower the heels 5 times. The legs remain bent throughout this exercise.

In plié position with the heels on the floor, lower one more inch. This is a great exercise for your thighs. Come back to plié position (knees bent). Lower one more inch and back to position 5 times.

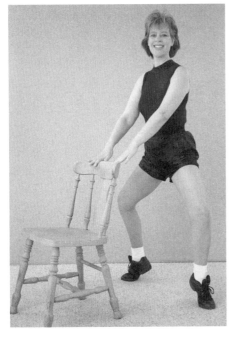

Kick Across

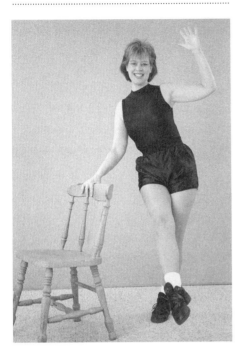

Our next two exercises emphasize aerobics. Aerobic exercises increase the capacities of your heart and lungs because you are moving your arms and legs at the same time. Feel free to keep one hand on the back of your chair to steady yourself.

Kick your right leg across in front of your supporting left leg. Then kick your left leg across the supporting right leg. Step and kick. Step and kick. Do this exercise for about 2 to 3 minutes, increasing as you build up stamina.

Walking in Place

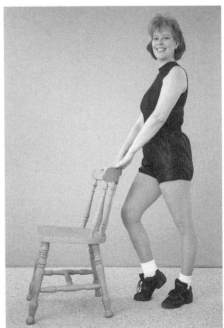

Your chair can serve as a walking machine—just stand behind it and hang on. Walk in place. You can do this for 2 to 5 minutes. As I suggested before, listen to music or talk on the telephone if you like. Aerobic exercise is more effective if you can walk and talk at the same time. It shows that you are not doing an exercise that is too strenuous for your body.

If you do not feel comfortable standing and walking but would like the benefits of an aerobic workout, do it sitting in your chair. Sit down and do the kick-across exercise and the walking exercise while sitting. Let your legs work.

Wall Push-Ups

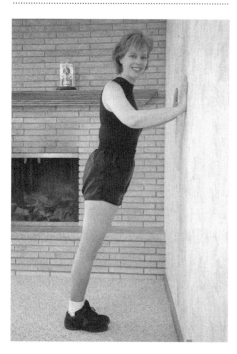

This is one of my favorite exercises. I have never felt great about my upper body strength, so doing push-ups on the floor was never quite comfortable. When something is not comfortable, we tend to avoid it, so that is what I did. When I discovered wall push-ups, I was delighted. I like how comfortable they feel, and I like how much fitter I feel.

Standing about a foot away from a sturdy wall, place your feet together. Place your hands about shoulder width apart on the wall at chest height. Keeping your body straight, lower yourself toward the wall. Bend from the ankle and stop just before you reach the wall. Now push back. I start with 10 push-ups. These are so comfortable that you might want to do 2, 3, or even 4 sets of 10 push-ups. Forty push-ups! Yes, it is possible.

Cool-Down — Look over the Shoulder

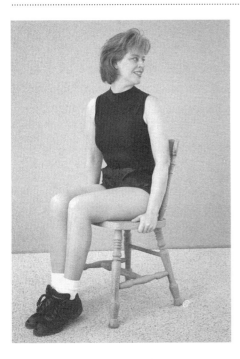

You may sit in your chair or remain standing for your cool-down. If you are standing, gently look over your shoulder toward the corner—or wall—behind you. Then, keeping your head level, turn to look over your other shoulder. Do this 3 times to each side. This will stretch your head and neck as well as give your back a gentle twist.

If you are sitting in your chair, as you turn to look over your shoulder, rest your arm on the back of your chair. This will give you a great backstretch. Hold your position, and do this exercise only twice to each side.

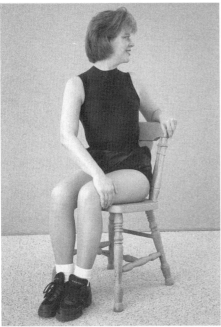

Lie on the Pillow

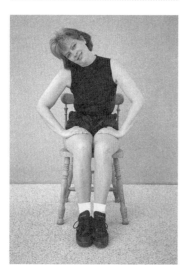

Gently lay your head on your right shoulder as if you were lying on a pillow. Now roll it down and up to an imaginary pillow on your left shoulder, then roll it down and back to the right side. Do this 3 times to each side. When doing neck exercises, please use caution. Take it slowly and very gently.

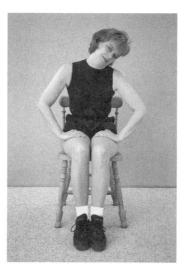

Big Mouth

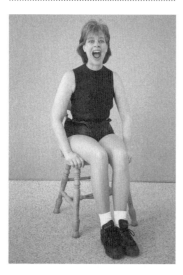

A wonderful way to relax and cool down is to do facial exercises. One of my favorites is Big Mouth. Relax your face. Now open your mouth as wide as you can and hold for 2 or 3 seconds. Close and relax. Open wide again! Do this 3 or 4 times. Relax. You have just completed Day Three.

One of the best ways to exercise is to play sports. It is fun and entertaining as well as a great workout—without you even thinking about what exactly your body is doing. Today we will have some fun. We will work out by imagining we are participating in different sports.

Warm-Up — Deep Breathing

Today we will try a deep breathing exercise that may challenge us. Do this exercise 2 to 3 times. First, inhale slowly, counting to 7. Then hold your breath for a count of 20 (I count fast). Then exhale to a count of 14. The exhale is the most challenging. Most people want to let all their air out in a second or two. Controlling the exhale helps to build up our lung capacity.

Throwing the Baseball

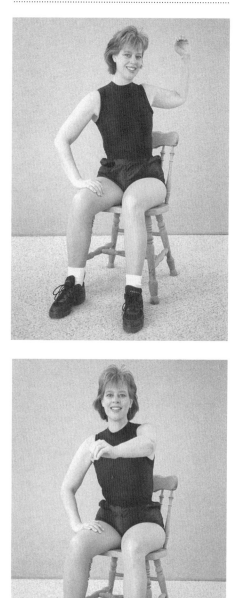

Sitting in your chair, imagine that you are throwing a ball to someone across the room. Bring your arm back and throw the ball. This is a great exercise. We just don't think of all the things our bodies do as we throw a ball. Throw with one arm 10 times, then do it 10 times with your other arm.

Batting

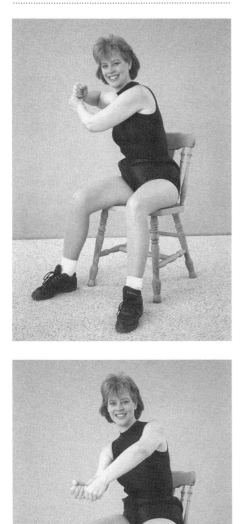

Now for batting practice—a great exercise for the waist and torso. Put an imaginary baseball bat in your hands, wiggle it a bit, then pull back and swing away. If you care to, you can hold a light weight as you swing (just don't let go!). Swing 10 times on one side, then switch to the other side and swing another 10 times.

Golf

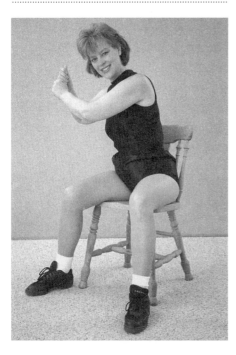

Sitting in your chair, let your feet part comfortably as if you were standing in front of your tee. Imagine that you will be swinging a golf club. This is a different type of swing than the baseball bat. Your hands start at about shoulder height, then the club swings down toward the ground and up. Swing your golf club 10 times one way, then switch to swinging from the other side.

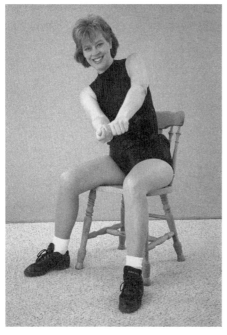

Basketball Free Throw

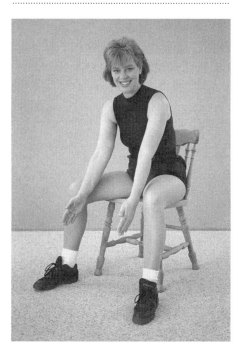

Few people probably remember this, but when I was young and learning to play basketball, the rules for girls were different from those for boys. The girls had to try a free throw with an underhand motion, not an overhand throw. Sitting in your chair with your feet flat on the floor and about shoulder-width apart, bring both arms down, between your knees, as if holding an imaginary ball. Bring the ball up and release. Bring your arms down, then throw and release about 10 times. This is a good exercise not only for your arms, but for your back as well.

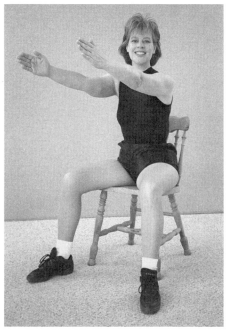

Soccer Kicks

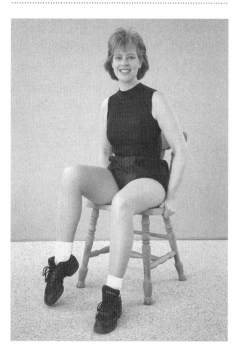

For this exercise you may sit in the chair or stand behind it. If sitting, imagine a soccer ball in front of you. Kick the ball, letting your leg swing from the knee 10 times. Then switch legs and kick 10 more times.

If you are standing, you may support yourself with your hand on the back of the chair. Kick the ball 10 times with one leg, then 10 times with the other.

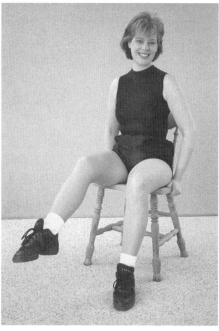

Boxing

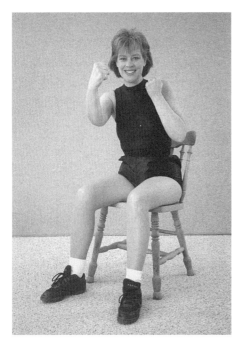

Boxing is a wonderful exercise, which works the upper body very effectively. We are going to do a series of punches. Make fists with your hands, with your thumbs resting outside the gripped fingers. Punch forward with your right hand 10 times, then punch forward with the left hand 10 times. Now alternate the hands. Right, left, right, left. Punch 10 times, take a short rest, then punch 10 more times. Put some strength into your punches by imagining yourself working out on a punching bag in a boxing gym.

Optional: You may continue your punching exercise by punching up rather than forward. Right hand, punch up 10 times. Left hand, up 10 times. Alternate 10 times.

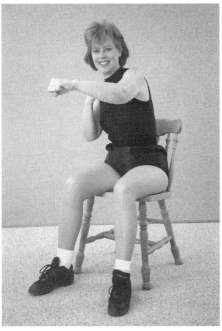

Swimming

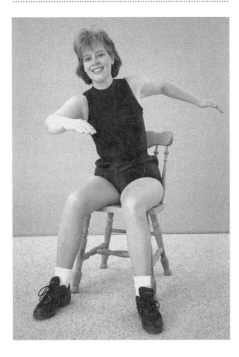

You can work out your arms and shoulders by swimming. Let's begin with a forward stroke. Use long arm motions as if doing the crawl, first right then left. Do this 10 times. Now let's stroke backward. Right back, left back. Do this 10 times. You'll soon notice the difference in the muscles exercised in the two movements.

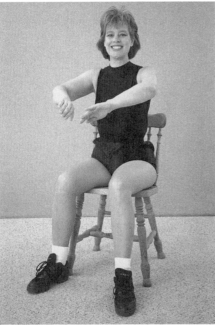

Now for the breaststroke. Your arms push forward in front of you then around to the side. Imagine the pressure of the water on your hands as you stroke. Stroke 10 times.

Bicycling

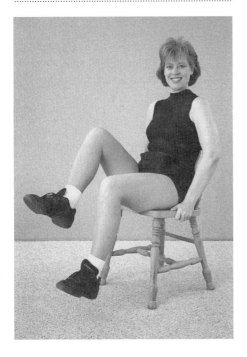

Sit back in your chair, holding on to the sides with your hands. Let your weight fall back on your hips so your legs can extend comfortably in front of you. Holding in your stomach muscles and being careful not to arch your back, pedal your legs as though on a bicycle or exercycle. This exercise will work not only your legs but also your stomach. Pedal for about a minute or two. If this becomes tedious, imagine the beautiful countryside you are riding through, or listen to some favorite music if you are at home. Oh, yes, remember to breathe.

Cool-Down

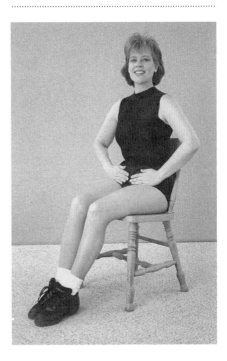

To cool down, take a nice tall stretch, reaching up with your arms and stretching out your legs. Now repeat your deep breathing exercise. Placing your hands on your stomach to feel your inhales and exhales, inhale for a count of 7. Hold for a count of 20. Exhale slowly to a count of 14. Repeat this breathing exercise twice more. You have successfully completed Day Four.

Some of you may want to exercise—or rather may have to exercise—in a public place where others are watching. Whether this is in your office or when you are on a train or airplane, you may feel uncomfortable if people know you are doing your exercises. So this day is for learning how to exercise without anyone knowing.

Deep Breathing

To begin, just take some deep breaths. Inhale slowly, hold for a few seconds, then exhale slowly. Do 3 to 5 deep breaths.

Hamstring Stretches

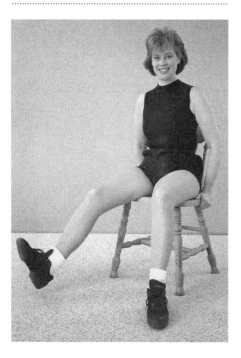

If you are sitting, extend your right leg slightly. Your leg need not be straight. Now pull your toes back so your foot is in a flexed position. This exercise is wonderful if you have a problem with leg cramps. Flex and relax the foot about 5 times, holding the flex position for a few seconds. Repeat with the left foot.

Shoulder Lifts and Rolls

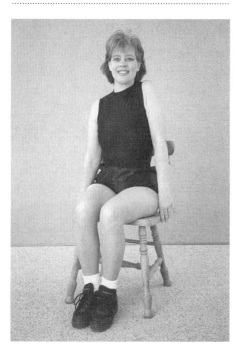

Slowly lift and lower your right shoulder 3 times. Now lift and lower your left shoulder 3 times. If you do this exercise slowly, no one will even notice.

Roll your right shoulder very slowly forward and around three times. Then roll it backward and around three times. Repeat both rolls with the left shoulder.

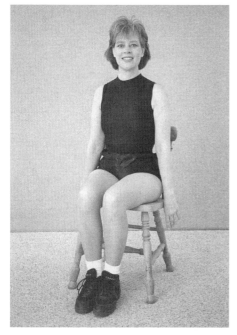

Release Move

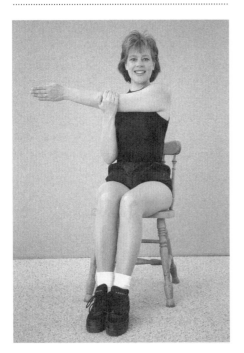

To gently relax your arms and shoulders—especially if you are hard at work at a desk job or sitting for a long time during travel—try this release move. With your left hand, grab your right elbow and pull your right arm across your body. Do the same for your left arm by grabbing your left elbow with your right hand and pulling your left arm across your body. Repeat once with each arm, holding the stretch for a few moments each time.

Walk Down the Chair

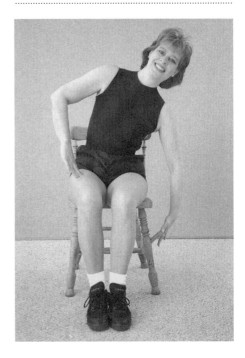

Sitting straight in your chair, let your fingers walk down the leg of the chair (see the picture at right) then let them walk back up. As your right hand walks, your left relaxes at your waist. Pretend that you are bending to pick up something. This exercise is for your waist, so keep your body facing straight forward, and you should feel a nice stretch in your left side. Repeat 4 or 5 more times on the right side, then 4 or 5 times on the left. Your feet should remain planted squarely on the floor without twisting to either side. Maintain normal breathing.

Ankle Circles

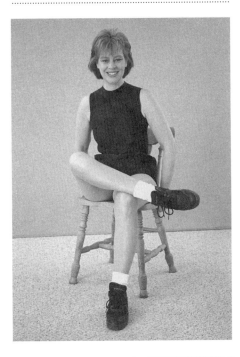

To exercise your ankles without attracting attention, let one leg cross naturally over the other. Now rotate the free ankle, circling slowly, first in one direction then the other. Before changing to the other leg, point and flex your foot, slowly emphasizing the point. Switch legs, and repeat the circles with the other ankle. Remember to slowly point and flex as well.

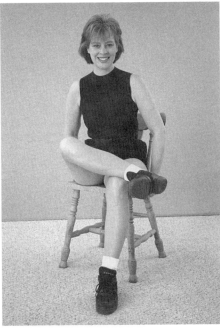

Stomach Isometrics

This exercise is wonderful and undetectable, so feel free to do it anytime and anyplace. Tighten your stomach muscles and hold, then relax. Do this at least 10 times. Exhale as you tighten your muscles. I like to hold for a little bit longer on the tenth one. This tightened feeling is what you want as you are doing other stomach exercises in the regular program, such as sit-ups, so concentrate on what it feels like.

Bottom Holds

This exercise is the isometric tightening of your behind. To do this effectively, you may want to get up out of your chair and casually stand someplace looking inconspicuous. Slowly tighten your bottom muscle. Hold. Now release. Repeat this tightening and relaxing for a total of 10 times. Again, I try to hold the last one a tad longer—just for good measure. This is great for times when you have to stand in line.

Wrist and Forearm Twists

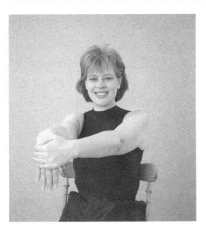

To warm up, gently grab the fingers of your right hand with your left, and push them back toward the wrist, both upward and downward. Now do the same to the left hand. You are now ready for the wrist and forearm twist.

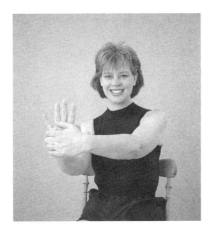

This exercise is normally done with weights, so you may want to hold something in your hands. Separately or at the same time, put your arms out in front of you. Hold your weights in your hands or make your hands into fists. Turn your wrists over

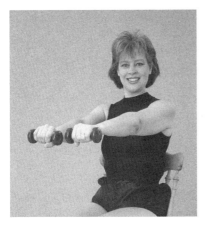

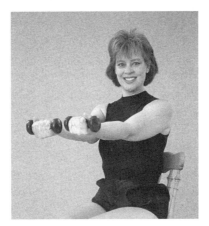

and back. Repeat this several times. The slower you do this and the tighter you grip your fists, the more you will feel the exercise work for you.

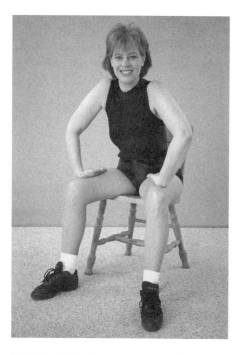

Another way to exercise your wrists is by sitting in your chair and placing your hands firmly on your knees. Now lean forward, pressing your elbows forward. Then, turning your hands over, place the backs of your hands on your knees and press your elbows back toward your body.

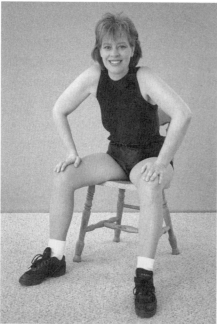

Back Stretch

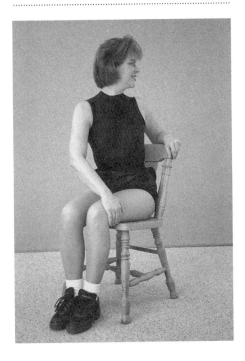

Very nonchalantly, turn in your chair, keeping your feet flat on the floor. Rest your arm on the back of your chair and look behind you. This will give you a nice back and torso twist. You may also feel a nice stretch in your neck and head. Now repeat to the other side, holding the stretch for just a few moments. Repeat to each side another time.

Cool-Down – Chin Jut

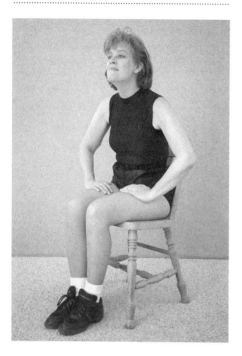

One of the best ways to relax and cool down after a workout is with face exercises. It feels so good!

Begin by letting your chin jut forward, then bring it back into a normal relaxed position. This might look a bit strange, so I recommend not to do this too many times if you are in a particularly crowded area or someone might get a bit worried about you. You will feel a nice stretch under your chin and along the front of your neck.

Eyebrows to the Ceiling

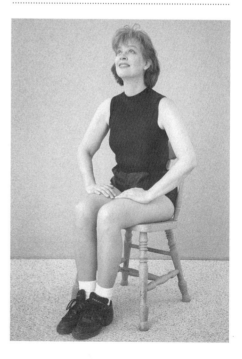

Let your eyes look up until you feel a stretch up through your cheek area and a wrinkling of your forehead. Repeat this exercise several times.

Smile and Pucker

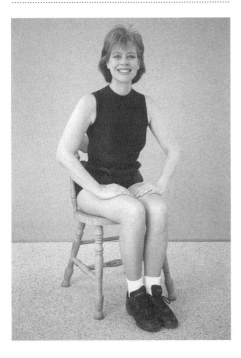

With your lips closed tightly, smile—a great, big smile. Hold, then pucker up for a big kiss. Big smile, big pucker. Repeat this until someone actually tries to kiss you on your pucker-up. Your face should feel very relaxed after you've completed these face exercises. You may even feel a little giggle welling up if you do them in front of a mirror.

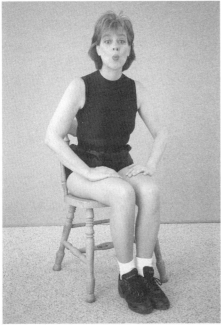

"Yes, Yes" Head

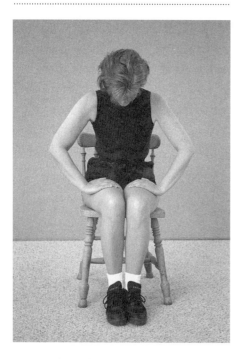

To complete your cool-down, slowly nod your head up and down as if saying, "yes, yes." You will find this is surprisingly relaxing.

The exercises during Day Five are inconspicuous and can be done almost anywhere. Do them during your workday, while waiting in traffic or in line, or in a crowded room. A boring lecture would be perfect for Day Five. Yes, you can do your exercises anyplace you'd like. Enjoy!

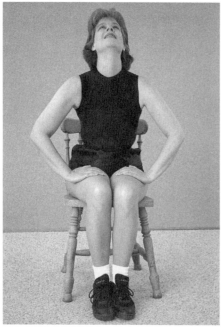

Chapter 4

Ten-Minute Miracles

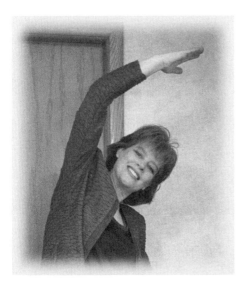

This chapter includes two ten-minute workouts, one for the person who is so busy that one simple workout is all they want or can handle, the other for the person who spends hours a day chained to a computer. Many people who are busy and organized already fit exercise into their daily schedule; if not, this short exercise sequence is a quickie that can be done anywhere and at any time. Exercise is especially important for very busy people because it keeps them balanced and energized as they move through their day.

The ten-minute workout for the computer user is a boon for anyone who spends long hours looking at a computer screen. Our eyes and hands, along with our backs and legs, get very tired from the repetitive action of inputting and the stiff position of our bodies at a desk. This may be the future for more and more of us, but our bodies were built to move. In addition to recharging and refreshing you, this ten-minute routine will protect you from stiff, sore muscles and tendonitis, along with eyestrain.

The good news is that it is possible to get fit even in these circumstances.

A Ten-Minute Miracle for the Truly Rushed

All of us have felt truly rushed at some time in our lives. Maybe some of you are truly rushed all the time. It feels as if there isn't a moment to spare—especially for exercise. We have all become aware in the past few years that taking the time for exercise, good nutrition, and a healthy lifestyle will keep us going for a good many more years than if we ignore these things. So here is a ten-minute workout that will cover all the bases.

Begin your workout with:

- Deep Breathing   page 8   3 reps

Continue warming up with:

- Overhead Stretch   page 9   4 reps each side
- Ankle Circles   page 20   4 reps each side
- Shoulder Swings   page 15   5 reps each side
- Side Twists   page 16   10 reps (5 each side)
- Stomach Isometrics   page 22   5 reps
- Bottom Holds   page 34   5 reps
- Isometric Thigh Closes (the Clam)   page 21   5 reps
- Grow Two Inches   page 34   3 reps
- Points and Lifts   pages 27–28   5 reps each side
- Plié   page 26   5 reps

Now select one of the Walking choices on page 31, but limit your walking time to 3–4 minutes.

Cool down with:

- Back Stretch   page 50   2 reps each side
- Head Stretches   pages 51–52

Finish with:

- Face Relaxation   pages 53–54   2 reps each exercise
- Deep Breathing   page 55   3 reps

■ Pointers for Making it Happen

If you still think you cannot find ten minutes to do all this at one time in your busy day here are a few pointers that might make your exercise program doable and productive.

You probably already know how to do more than one thing at a time—maybe even three or four things at the same time. So what I am going to suggest is that you exercise while you are doing something else. Do your stretches and warm-ups when you wake up in the morning, before you get out of bed. Or you can do them in the kitchen while you're making coffee.

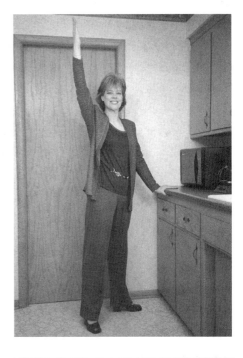

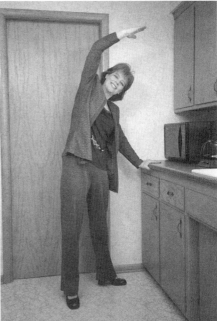

A Ten-Minute Miracle for the Truly Rushed

The Stomach Isometrics and the Bottom Holds are ideal to do while you are brushing your teeth. Or try them in the shower.

You can do an Isometric Thigh Close (The Clam) in your kitchen, or in your car. Try pointing and flexing your feet as you get in or out of your car. These will be great for your thighs, arms, and ankles. Many of these exercises are great for doing in the car. It's better than talking on your cell phone—or maybe you can do that at the same time, too!

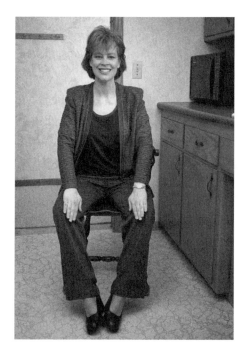

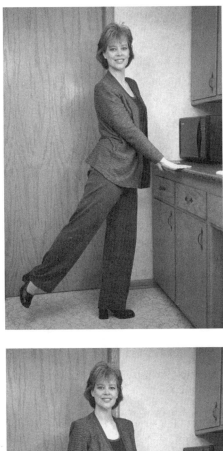

After a hard day, you'll love doing the Cool-Down exercises as you watch the nightly news or the late, late movie. You can also do these right in your bed. The Back Stretch, the Head Stretches, and the Face Relaxation are restful and feel wonderful. Just the thing for the end of a stressful but productive day. They get you ready for sleep and for tomorrow. And always finish with more Deep Breathing.

For additional places to exercise, consider these:

- Grow Two Inches while you wait for the elevator

- Points and Lifts and Pliés as you wait for your dinner to microwave or as you make your coffee

- Weight Exercises: Several people have told me their secrets for getting in their weight exercises. One idea is placing the weights next to the washer and drier so you can exercise as you wait to put clothes in and take them out. What a great idea!

■ Combinations

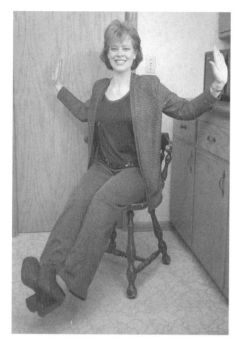

Another suggestion for the truly rushed is to combine exercises. Do several of them at the same time. Here are some combinations that work well:

- Combine the Ankle exercises found on pages 19 and 20 with Arm exercises such as Circles (page 12), Crisscross (page 14), and Shoulder Swings (page 15).

- Do Waist exercises like the Side Twist (page 16) as you do your Walking and Kicks (pages 31 and 33).

- As you do Leg Lifts (page 23) for your stomach, do your Ankles All-Position Stretch (page 19) and add a few Curls (page 38) or Punches (page 49) for your arms.

Walk whenever and wherever you can, adding a few arm movements. Use any of the exercises shown with weights beginning on page 37 as arm exercises—minus the weights. Because you are already busy and rushed, walk faster. I do not suggest that you run if your focus is low-impact exercise. Walking quickly will get you there just as fast and will allow you to exercise at the same time.

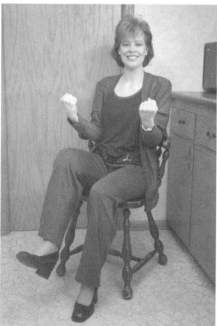

In this age of computers, many of us find ourselves glued to the keyboard and screen more than we would like to be—at least more than our bodies would like to be. Some areas of our body need special attention when we are computer bound for many hours at a time. Here are a few exercises that will help you through a long day.

Hands

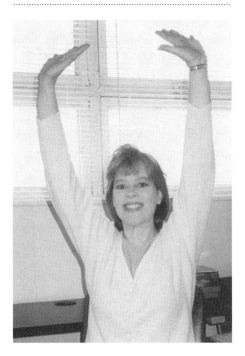

Hands and fingers that begin to feel stiff and sore will benefit from these special exercises. Begin by stretching your hands—fingers spread—above your head. If you are in a situation that would make you feel uncomfortable holding your arms above your head with your fingers stretched, push back your chair and stretch your arms in front of you. Hold the stretch, feeling your arms and fingers lengthen.

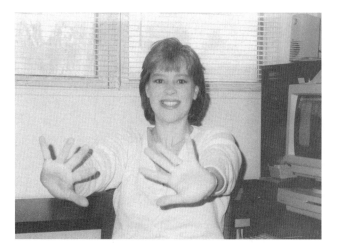

Wrists

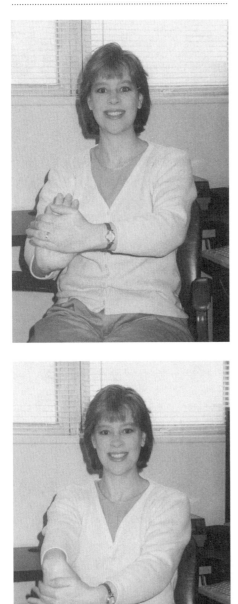

Now gently press your wrist back toward your arm by pushing with your left hand against your right upper palm. Repeat this with the right hand pressing on the left upper palm. With the left hand, press the right hand toward the underside of the wrist by gently pushing on the back of the right hand. Repeat this, pressing with the right hand on the back of the left. This will stretch your wrists. These exercises are also shown on page 66.

Fingers

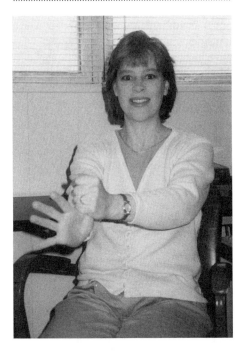

This finger exercise is also shown on page 67. Grasping hold of each finger on your right hand with the left, gently stretch the middle of each finger. Do the same for the fingers on the left hand. Now gently stretch the knuckle of each finger as well as the joint close to the fingertip.

Head and Neck

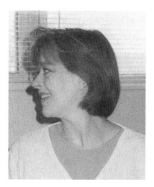

When you sit at the computer, your head and neck are areas that need extra attention. Begin by looking over your shoulder to the back corner of the room. Turn to the other side and look over the other shoulder. Then gently nod your head up and down "yes, yes." Turn your head from side to side as if saying "no, no." Lay your head on your right shoulder as if on a pillow, then lay it on your left shoulder. For additional neck exercises, look at pages 51–52.

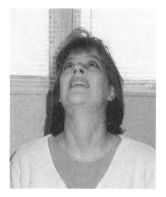
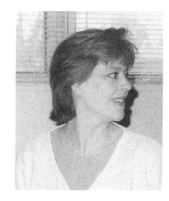
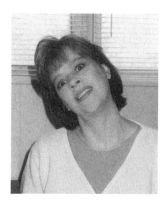

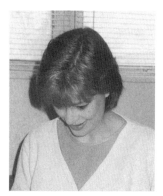
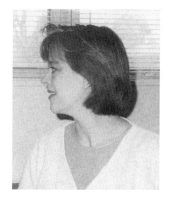
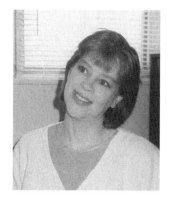

The back takes the brunt of the abuse from sitting too long at a computer. A few back exercises every hour will certainly improve your physical situation as well as your mental attitude.

Back Twists

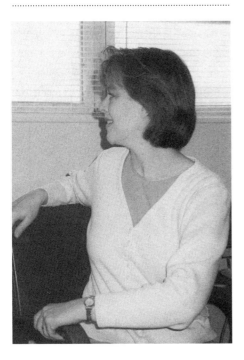

Begin with your feet flat on the floor and your knees and hips facing forward. Turn at the waist, placing your right arm across the back of your chair (hopefully your chair back is not too high). Place your left hand on the arm or side of the chair, allowing your back to feel a comfortable stretch. Now do the same once to the other side.

Modified Toe Touch

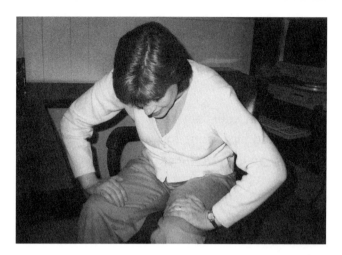

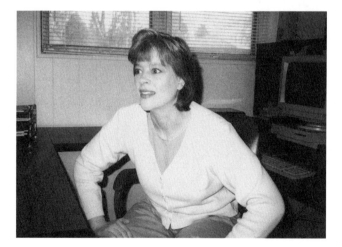

On page 10 you will see the Modified Toe Touch. This is an excellent exercise for the back. Placing your hands on your knees, wrists outward, to support your weight, lean forward so your elbows stick out to the sides. Drop your head and round your back. Now lift your head and straighten your back, being careful not to arch it. Repeat this exercise several times. Round, straighten. Round, straighten.

Shoulder Rolls and Lifts

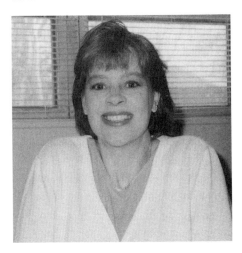

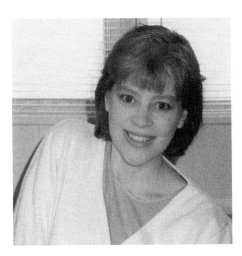

Come up to a straight but relaxed sitting position and allow your shoulders to roll back and around. Repeat the roll back and around. Reverse directions, rolling the shoulders forward and around. Slowly lift your right shoulder up and let it drop. Up, then drop. Now lift the left shoulder up and let it drop. Repeat.

Sitting at a computer for any length of time can be stressful. And whenever we feel stress, our faces are likely to show it. On pages 53–54 you will find a number of face relaxation exercises that will feel wonderful if you begin to feel stress from staring into a computer screen.

Big Mouth

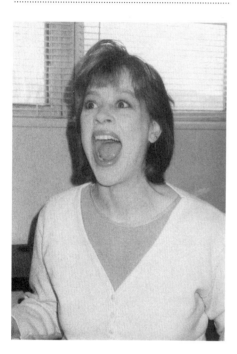

The first one I would suggest would be Big Mouth. Begin by relaxing your facial muscles. Now stretch your mouth open as wide as you can, showing your teeth and making a big mouth. Then relax. Open wide. Relax. Repeat 3–4 times.

Chin Jut

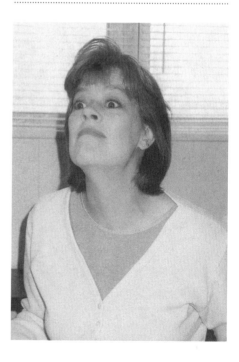

Push your chin forward as far as you can. You should feel a stretch in your jaw and front neck muscles. Relax, then jut your chin out again, and hold the position. Relax. You may want to repeat this several times.

Other exercises that feel great to a computer user are the ankle exercises found on pages 19 and 20. Stretch your legs out, and do the four position stretches, then, placing your ankle on your knee, gently rotate your ankle. Before switching to the other leg, lift your supporting leg up and down with the ankle still resting across the knee.

The Stomach Isolations found on page 23 are great to do not only as you take this exercise break but also as you work at the computer. Tighten your stomach muscles, then relax. Do several of these, holding longer each time.

One reason we feel the need for exercises to relieve stiffness while sitting at a computer is because of the way our body is positioned at the desk. Place your feet squarely on the floor so as not to allow your body to lean to one side or the other. Often people will cross their legs at their desk or sit lopsided, putting all their weight in one area. Sitting properly will relieve some of the problems we feel. Try the Grow Two Inches exercise found on page 34 while sitting at your chair. This will allow you to stretch to a nice straight posture. Then, holding in your stomach, as we just did with our Isolations, will allow us to keep that posture. If you feel rigid at first, practice until this position becomes straight yet relaxed. Then do your Deep Breathing (page 55). Your day at the computer will feel much less stressful.

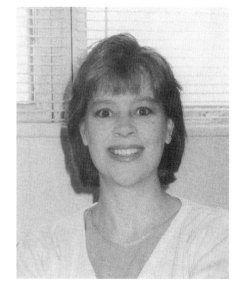

Additional Reading

When you are ready to progress to a more intense program try:

Jane Fonda Workout Book, by Jane Fonda. New York: Simon and Schuster, 1981.

Check out the many videos recommended in *Fitness for Dummies,* by Suzanne Schlosberg and Liz Newporent. Foster City, CA, Chicago, IL, Southlake, TX: IDG Books Worldwide, 1996.

For additional information about fitness:

Fit or Fat?, by Covert Bailey. Boston: Houghton Mifflin, 1978.

The Fit or Fat Woman, by Covert Bailey and Lea Bishop. Boston: Houghton Mifflin, 1989.

For additional information about arthritis and osteoporosis:

Maximizing the Arthritis Cure, by Jason Theodosakis. New York: St. Martin's Press, 1998.

The Arthritis Cure, by Jason Theodosakis. New York: St. Martin's Press, 1997

Care of the Older Adult, by Joan M. Birchenall and Mary Eileen Streight. Philadelphia: J. B. Lippincott, 1993.

Alternative Medicine, by the Burton Goldberg Group. Tiburon, CA: Future Medicine Publishing, 1997.

Appendix: Easy Exercise Checklist

After you have gone through and selected the exercise plan that best fits your lifestyle and time frame, you will gradually become familiar and comfortable with the explanation and illustrations included with each exercise. The Easy Exercise Checklist is designed to help you with your fitness progress at this point. It lists all the exercises for the One-Hour Program and the "But I Don't Have Time..." Program, with a recommended number of beginning repetitions. The warm-up exercises and cooldowns may remain the same throughout your exercise program because they are meant for just that—warming up and cooling down. For the remainder of the exercises I have recommended an "increase to" goal to strive for. This is listed in the "Goal" column. If you are doing really well you may wish to increase beyond this number, and that is your personal choice. You also may wish to add repetitions to your cooldown if you have increased your workout significantly or feel the need for an additional stretch after your walking.

On the right side of the checklist is a place for you to check off the exercise when it is completed. There are five check-off columns. You may wish to use these to chart your progress with your program, and date your workouts. Or you can simply use them as an aid to keep your place as you go through your workout.

Feel free to copy these sheets if you find them a useful aid for your fitness program. This checklist is also perfect to carry with you as you travel, or if you are using this program at your workplace. A quick glance will help you run through your workout more efficiently and at a comfortable pace.

Appendix: Easy Exercise Checklist

ONE-HOUR PROGRAM—EXERCISE	PAGE	RECOMMENDED REPS	INCREASE TO — GOAL	X	X	X	X	X
WARM-UP								
1. Deep breathing	8	3 times						
2. Overhead stretch	9	Hold 5 counts						
3. Modified toe touch	10	3 times						
4. Shoulder rolls and lifts	11	4 directions / 2 each side						
5. Hamstring stretch	11	2 / each leg						
ARMS								
1. Circles	12	16 / each direction						
2. Windshield wipers	13	16 times						
Release move	13							
3. Crisscross	14	3 / on 3 sides						
Release move	14							
4. Shoulder swings	15	4 directions / 2 each side						
WAIST								
1. Side twists	16	16 times						
2. Combination	17	4 / each side						
3. Walk down the chair	18	8 counts down						
		8 counts up / each side						
4. Wall pushes	18	8 counts / each side						
ANKLES								
1. All-position stretch	19	5 times						
2. Ankle circles	20	Need not count						
INNER THIGHS								
1. Bent leg lifts	21	10 / each side	20 / each side					
2. Isometric thigh closes (The Clam)	21	5 counts / 2 times						

Appendix: Easy Exercise Checklist

ONE-HOUR PROGRAM—EXERCISE	PAGE	RECOMMENDED REPS	INCREASE TO — GOAL	X	X	X	X	X
STOMACH								
1. Stomach isometrics	22	10 times						
2. Chair sit-ups	23	10 times	20 times					
3. Leg lifts	23	Varies						
AEROBIC WARM-UP								
1. Hamstring stretch	25	Hold stretch						
Heel lift	25	5 times						
One inch lower	25	5 times						
2. Plié	26	5 times						
One inch lower	26	5 times						
Heel lift	26	5 times						
3. Points and lifts—1	27	5 / each side						
Points and lifts—2	28	5 / each side						
4. Adding arm movement 1	29	5 minutes						
Adding arm movement 2	30	5 minutes						
5. Walking	31	20 minutes						
AEROBIC COOL-DOWN								
1. Hamstring stretch	32	8 counts / each side						
2. Bottom kicks	33	10 / each leg	20 / each leg					
3. Back leg lifts	33	10 / each leg	20 / each leg					
4. Bottom holds	34	10 counts						
5. Grow two inches	34	5 times						
6. Wall push-ups	35	10 times	20 / 30 / 40					
OPTIONAL COOL-DOWN								
Repeat plié	36	5 times						
Repeat hamstring stretch	36	2 / each leg						

Appendix: Easy Exercise Checklist

ONE-HOUR PROGRAM— EXERCISE	PAGE	RECOMMENDED REPS	INCREASE TO — GOAL	X	X	X	X	X
WEIGHTS								
1. Curls	38	2 sets / 8 reps each 3 sets / 10 reps each	2 sets / 10 reps each					
2. Windshield wipers	39	2 sets / 8 reps each	2 sets / 10 reps each					
3. Weed puller	40	2 sets / 8 reps each 3 sets / 10 reps each	2 sets / 10 reps each					
4. Magnetic pectoral pulls	41	2 sets / 8 reps 3 sets / 10 reps	2 sets / 10 reps					
5. Kissing weights	42	2 sets / 8 reps 3 sets / 10 reps	2 sets / 10 reps					
Release move 1	43	Varies						
Release move 2	43	Varies						
Release move 3	44	Varies						
6. Waist stretches	45	8 / each side						
7. Side and forward lifts	46	8 / each side / 2 directions						
8. Triceps lift	47	2 sets / 8 reps 3 sets / 10 reps	2 sets / 10 reps					
9. Wrist and forearm twists	48	2 sets / 8 reps	2 sets / 10 reps					
10. Final punches	49	2 sets / 8 reps						
Release move	49							
COOL-DOWN								
1. Back stretch	50	2 / each side						
2. Head stretches	51							
Look over shoulder	51	2 / each side						
Up and down	51	2 times						
Pillow rest	52	2 each side						
Shoulder to shoulder	52	2 each side						
"No, no"	52	2 each side						

Appendix: Easy Exercise Checklist

ONE-HOUR PROGRAM—EXERCISE	PAGE	RECOMMENDED REPS	INCREASE TO — GOAL	X	X	X	X	X
COOL-DOWN (cont.)								
3. Face relaxation	53							
Chin jut	53	As desired						
Eyebrow rise	53	As desired						
Smile and pucker	54	As desired						
Big mouth	54	As desired						
4. Deep breathing	55	Inhale 7 counts						
		Hold 20 counts						
		Exhale 14 counts						
5. Total relaxation	56							

"BUT I DON'T HAVE TIME …" PROGRAM	PAGE	RECOMMENDED REPS	INCREASE TO — GOAL	X	X	X	X	X
DAY 1: START DAY								
1. Warm-up/ deep breathing	72	3 times						
2. Shoulder rolls and swings	73	3 shrugs						
	73	3 rolls forward 3 rolls back						
	73	3 giant swings forward / each arm 3 giant swings back / each arm						
3. Waist twists	74	6 times						
4. Ankle stretches	75	Point / flex / 5 times						
	75	Roll / 5 times / both directions						
5. Leg lifts	76	10 / each leg	20 / each leg					

Appendix: Easy Exercise Checklist

"BUT I DON'T HAVE TIME ..." PROGRAM	PAGE	RECOMMENDED REPS	INCREASE TO — GOAL	X	X	X	X	X
DAY 1: START DAY (cont.)								
6. Arms								
Curls	77	8 reps (each side or together)	2 sets / 8 reps					
Side lifts	78	8 reps	2 sets / 8 reps					
7. Bottom kicks	79	10 times / each leg						
Side leg lifts	79	10 times / each leg						
8. Cool-Down								
Round back	80	5 times						
Head rolls	80	5 times / each side						
Deep breathing	80	3–5 times						
DAY 2: I CAN DO IT AGAIN DAY								
1. Warm-up—overhead stretch	81	Hold Pulse 6–8 times						
2. Arms—little circles	82	10 times	20 times / 30 times					
3. Wall pushes	83	10 times / each side						
4. Ankle circles and lifts	84	8 times 2 directions / each leg						
Lower leg lifts	84	3–5 times						
5. The clam	85	2 sets / 8 counts						
6. Chair sit-ups	85	10 times	20 times / 30 times					
7. Triceps lift	86	2 sets / 8 times						
8. Magnetic pectoral pulls	87	2 sets / 8 times						
9. Cool-down								
Shoulder lifts	88	Lift / 3 times each side Roll forward / 3 times each side Roll backward / 3 times each side						

Appendix: Easy Exercise Checklist

"BUT I DON'T HAVE TIME ..." PROGRAM	PAGE	RECOMMENDED REPS	INCREASE TO — GOAL	X	X	X	X	X
DAY 2: I CAN DO IT AGAIN DAY (cont.)								
No, no head	89							
Deep breathing	89	3–5 times						
DAY 3: WALKING DAY								
1. Grow two inches	90	5 times						
2. Hamstring stretch	91	8 times Lift / 5 times each leg 1 inch more / 5 times each leg						
3. Points and lifts	92	Point side / 5 times each leg						
	92	Point and kick side / 5 times each leg						
	92	Point and lift back / 5 times each leg						
	92	Point back / 5 times each leg						
4. Front and back leg swings	93	5 times						
5. Pliés	94	5 times						
Lift heels	94	5 times						
One inch more	94	5 times						
6. Kick across	95	2–3 minutes						
7. Walking in place	95	2–5 minutes						
8. Wall push-ups	96	10 times	20, 30, 40 times					
9. Cool-down								
Look over the shoulder	97	3 times / each side						
Lie on the pillow	98	3 times / each side						
Big mouth	98	3–4 times						

"BUT I DON'T HAVE TIME ..." PROGRAM	PAGE	RECOMMENDED REPS	INCREASE TO — GOAL	X	X	X	X	X
DAY 4: SPORTS DAY								
1. Deep breathing	99	2–3 times Inhale / 7 counts Hold / 20 counts Exhale / 14 counts						
2. Throwing the baseball	100	10 times / each arm						
Batting	101	10 times / each side						
3. Golf	102	10 times / each side						
4. Basketball free throw	103	10 times						
5. Soccer kicks	104	10 times / each leg						
6. Boxing	105	10 / each arm 10 / alternate						
optional / punching upward	105	10 / each arm 10 / alternate						
7. Swimming	106	10 forward / each arm 10 back / each arm 10 breast stroke						
8. Bicycling	107	1–2 minutes						
9. Cool-down— deep breathing	107	Same count as above						
DAY 5: INCONSPICUOUS EXERCISES								
1. Deep breathing	108	3–5 times						
2. Hamstring stretches	108	5 times each leg						
3. Shoulder lifts and rolls	109	Lift / 3 times each Roll forward / 3 times each Roll backward / 3 times each						
4. Release move	110	1 time / each arm						
5. Walk down the chair	110	4–5 times each side						

Appendix: Easy Exercise Checklist

"BUT I DON'T HAVE TIME ..." PROGRAM	PAGE	RECOMMENDED REPS	INCREASE TO — GOAL	X	X	X	X	X
DAY 5: INCONSPICUOUS EXERCISES (cont.)								
6. Ankle circles	111	Varies						
7. Stomach isometrics	112	10 times						
8. Bottom holds	112	10 times						
9. Wrist and forearm twists	113	Varies						
10. Back stretch	115	2 times / each side						
11. Cool-down – face relaxation								
Chin jut	116	Varies						
Eyebrows to the ceiling	116	Varies						
Smile and pucker	117	Varies						
"Yes, yes" head	118	Varies						

EXERCISE / HEALTH

TREAT YOUR BACK WITHOUT SURGERY: The Best Non-Surgical Alternatives for Eliminating Back and Neck Pain *by* Stephen Hochschuler, M.D., and Bob Reznik

Eighty percent of back pain sufferers can get well without surgery. This guide discusses a range of non-surgical techniques — from Tai Chi and massage therapy to chiropractic treatment and acupuncture — as well as exercise plans, diet and stress management techniques, and tips to ease everyday pain. Because surgery is sometimes necessary, you'll also get advice on how to find the best surgeon and what questions to ask.

224 pages ... 52 illus. ... Paperback $14.95

RECOVERING FROM BREAST SURGERY: Exercises to Strengthen Your Body and Relieve Pain *by* Diana Stumm, P.T.

Many women find that breast surgery leaves them with crippling pain. Physical therapist Diana Stumm has worked with women recovering from breast surgery for many years and explains how to recuperate and recover mobility. With warmth and understanding, she discusses the best exercises for mastectomy, lumpectomy, radiation, reconstruction, and lymphedema. Using clear drawings, she describes a program of specific stretches, massage techniques, and general exercises that form the crucial steps to a full and pain-free recovery.

128 pages ... 25 illus. ... Paperback ... $11.95

ONCE A MONTH: Understanding and Treating PMS *by* Katharina Dalton, M.D.

Once considered an imaginary complaint, PMS has at last received the serious attention it deserves, thanks largely to the work of Dr. Katharina Dalton. Premenstrual syndrome may in fact be the world's most common condition: surveys show that as many as 75% of women experience at least one symptom. The sixth edition of this classic book addresses the whole range of possible treatments — from self-care methods such as the three-hour starch diet and relaxation techniques to the newest medical options, including updated guidelines for progesterone therapy.

320 pages ... 55 illus. ... Paperback ... $15.95 ... 6th edition

MACULAR DEGENERATION: Living Positively with Vision Loss *by* Betty Wason and James J. McMillan, M.D.

Age-related macular degeneration (AMD) is an affliction of progressive vision loss and is the leading cause of legal blindness for people over the age of 50. Betty Wason contracted this eye disease and together with Dr. James McMillan offers readers a complete resource for people with AMD and their families. Topics include: what happens to the eye as a result of AMD, how to choose a doctor, diet and food supplements that can help, high-tech and low-tech products that can help with everyday activities, and the important role of family members.

256 pages ... 10 illus. ... Paperback $13.95

WOMEN'S HEALTH / NUTRITION

HER HEALTHY HEART: A Woman's Guide to Preventing and Reversing Heart Disease Naturally *by* Linda Ojeda, Ph.D.

Heart disease is the #1 killer of women. Linda Ojeda, Ph.D., bestselling author of *Menopause Without Medicine*, gives women the facts about this disease and describes ways they can prevent it naturally. She discusses nutrition factors and what women can do to modify their diet to benefit their heart. Individual chapters discuss fat, fiber, protein, B-vitamins, and antioxidants. Finally Ojeda discusses lifestyle changes such as managing stress and taking the time to enjoy life.

352 pages ... 7 illus. ... Paperback $14.95

MENOPAUSE WITHOUT MEDICINE *by* Linda Ojeda, Ph.D.

Linda Ojeda broke new ground when she began her study of nonmedical approaches to menopause more than ten years ago. In this update of her classic book, she discusses natural sources of estrogen; how mood swings are affected by diet and personality; and the newest research on osteoporosis, breast cancer, and heart disease. She thoroughly examines the hormone therapy debate; suggests natural remedies for depression, hot flashes, sexual changes, and skin and hair problems. **As seen in *Time* magazine.**

352 pages ... 40 illus. ... Paperback $14.95 ... Hard cover $23.95 ... 3rd edition

THE NATURAL ESTROGEN DIET: Healthy Recipes for Perimenopause and Menopause *by* Dr. Lana Liew with Linda Ojeda, Ph.D.

To manage the symptoms of menopause, doctors are prescribing hormone replacement therapy (HRT) at record levels. Recent studies, however, show that increasing the natural estrogen in the diet can successfully manage menopause.

Here, two women's health and nutrition experts offer women more than 100 easy and delicious recipes to naturally increase their level of estrogen. Each recipe includes nutritional information such as the calories, cholesterol, and calcium content. The authors also provide an overview of how phytoestrogens (plant estrogen) work, which foods contain the highest levels of natural estrogen, and how to approach a natural estrogen diet successfully. A general health plan for women forms an important part of the book emphasizing preventative measures and encouraging good health practices.

224 pages ... Paperback ... $13.95

FAD-FREE NUTRITION *by* Fredrick J. Stare, M.D., Ph.D., and Elizabeth M. Whelan, Sc.D., M.P.H.

The media is flooded with claims of quick-fix nutritional nirvanas. Using up-to-date nutrition information and basing their approach on sound scientific principles and legitimate studies, the authors help the reader sort fact from fiction. They debunk claims that the food supply is irreversibly tainted, that disease is an inevitable result of eating, that nutritional supplements are a necessity, and that food technology is employed against the public interest.

256 pages ... Paperback ... $14.95

Prices subject to change

HEALTH

COMPUTER RESOURCES FOR PEOPLE WITH DISABILITIES *by* the
Alliance for Technology Access

Computer technologies offer dramatic possibilties for people with disabilities —
disabilities ranging from sight and mobility to learning, reading, and
understanding. This acclaimed book helps them access today's technology to
achieve goals and change lives.

Written by a group of practicing experts in the field, this step-by-step guide to
approaching computer innovations ahs been carefully updated.

**"This book offers something not other does: a guide to maneuvering
the growing world of computers, both the mainstream and the assistive
technology, to find what is right for you." — Stephen Hawking, from
the Foreword**

288 pages ... Paperback $17.95 ... Hard cover $27.95

**THE PLEASURE PRESCRIPTION: To Love, to Work, to Play — Life in the
Balance** *by* Paul Pearsall, Ph.D.   *New York Times Bestseller!*

This bestselling book is a prescription for stressed-out lives. Dr. Pearsall
maintains that contentment, wellness, and long life can be found by devoting
time to family, helping others, and slowing down to savor life's pleasures.

Current wisdom suggests that anything that tastes, smells, or feels good can't
be good for us. "That's plain wrong," says Dr. Pearsall, a leading proponent of
the relationship between pleasure, stress, the immune system, and brain
chemistry. "Balanced pleasure is the natural way to physical and mental health."

"This book will save your life." — Montel Williams

288 pages ... Paperback $13.95 ... Hard cover $23.95 ... Audio $16.95

**WRITE YOUR OWN PLEASURE PRESCRIPTION: 60 Ways to Create
Balance & Joy in Your Life** *by* Paul Pearsall, Ph.D.

In *The Pleasure Prescription* (see above), Dr. Pearsall explained these
life-changing lessons. For the many readers who have written since asking for
ways to translate the harmony of Oceanic life to their own lives, he offers this
companion volume. It is full of ideas for bringing the spirit of aloha — the ability
to fully connect with oneself and with others — to everyday life.

Pearsall emphasizes that pleasure is balance, healthy balance. He encourages
readers to disengage from the headlong rush and frenzy of Western life in order
to feel the pleasure that comes from a calm acceptance of the world around us
and the connection we have with others. From learning how to "go with how it
goes" at work (pleasure prescripton #18) to "just say maybe" (pleasure
prescription #26) Pearsall's fun, profound, and caring suggestions enable
people to shift their lives so that they feel the deep joy that can be part of
each day.

224 pages ... Paperback ... $12.95

ORDER FORM

10% DISCOUNT on orders of $50 or more –
20% DISCOUNT on orders of $150 or more –
30% DISCOUNT on orders of $500 or more –
On cost of books for fully prepaid orders

NAME

ADDRESS

CITY/STATE   ZIP/POSTCODE

PHONE   COUNTRY

TITLE	QTY	PRICE	TOTAL
Get Fit While You Sit		@ $12.95	
Treat Your Back Without Surgery		@ $14.95	
Recovering from Breast Surgery		@ $11.95	
Once a Month		@ $15.95	
Please list other titles below:			
		@ $	
		@ $	
		@ $	
		@ $	
		@ $	
		@ $	

Shipping costs
First book: $3.00 by book post; $4.50 by UPS or to ship outside the U.S.
Each additional book: $1.00
For rush orders and bulk shipments call us at (800) 266-5592

SUBTOTAL	
Less discount @ _____ %	(_____)
TOTAL COST OF BOOKS	
Calif. residents add sales tax	
Shipping & handling	
TOTAL ENCLOSED	
Please pay in U.S. funds only	

❑ Check ❑ Money Order ❑ Visa ❑ M/C ❑ Discover

Card # _____ Exp date _____

Signature _____

Complete and mail to:
Hunter House Inc., Publishers
PO Box 2914, Alameda CA 94501-0914
Orders: 1-800-266-5592 . . . ordering@hunterhouse.com
Phone (510) 865-5282 Fax (510) 865-4295
❑ Check here to receive our FREE book catalog

GFW 5/98